MAY CONTAIN ANXIETY

May Contain Anxiety

Managing the Overwhelm of Parenting Children with Food Allergies

Tamara Hubbard, MA, LCPC

Johns Hopkins University Press
Baltimore

Printed in the United States of America on acid- free paper
9 8 7 6 5 4 3 2 1

Johns Hopkins University Press
2715 North Charles Street
Baltimore, Maryland 21218
www.press.jhu.edu

Library of Congress Cataloging-in-Publication Data is available.

A catalog record for this book is available from the British Library.
ISBN 978-1-4214-4957-9 (hardcover)
ISBN 978-1-4214-4958-6 (paperback)
ISBN 978-1-4214-4959-3 (ebook)

A catalog record for this book is available from the British Library.

Special discounts are available for bulk purchases of this book.
For more information, please contact Special Sales at specialsales@jh.edu.

EU GPSR Authorized Representative
LOGOS EUROPE, 9 rue Nicolas Poussin, 17000, La Rochelle, France
E-mail: Contact@logoseurope.eu

To my husband and my boys—you are my world.
And to all the families managing allergies—you've got this!

CONTENTS

Introduction: Are You Ready to Feel Less Overwhelmed About Parenting a Child with Allergies? *1*

1. Exploring Unhelpful Allergy Parenting Narratives *20*

2. Recognizing Common Allergy Parenting Traps *43*

3. Setting Developmentally Focused Allergy Parenting Goals *70*

4. Responding Differently to Anxious Thoughts *103*

5. Focusing on All That Matters—Not Just Allergy Safety *130*

6. Developing Flexible Perspectives on Allergy Parenting *154*

7. Putting Your Balanced, Mindful Allergy Parenting Plan into Action *181*

Notes *207*
Resources *217*
Acknowledgements *225*
Index *229*

Introduction

Are You Ready to Feel Less Overwhelmed About Parenting a Child with Allergies?

For parents, there are days that are etched in your mind forever. The days your children were born. Their first words and first steps. Their first days of school. But when you're the parent of a child diagnosed with an allergic condition, you've got another memory etched in your mind: the day you received the diagnosis and joined the Allergy Parenting Club. In an instant, it feels as though your world has been turned upside down and that everything you anticipated for your child's future is no longer possible—at least, not in the way you envisioned it. You think about how they won't be able to effortlessly attend birthday parties, enjoy the same foods as others, get through colds without asthma attacks, and travel safely. Then there's the worst fear of all—wondering if your child will experience an allergic reaction or asthma attack that might take their life. These worries, especially the latter, make you feel so overwhelmed that it's hard to see straight and envision what life will look like for your child and for you as an allergy parent.

WHY I WROTE THIS BOOK

So, why did I write this book? Because I'm not just a licensed therapist who works with allergy parents. I'm also a member of the Allergy Parenting Club and have been since 2012. Like you, I never envisioned myself being in this club since no one in my family had food allergies. Nonetheless, here I am, and therefore, I know firsthand how hard this journey can be. How an allergy diagnosis turns your world upside down in an instant. How fear, anxiety, and constant "what-if" thoughts can send you on an emotional rollercoaster, sometimes on a daily (or hourly) basis. How raising a child with an allergic disease can throw your mind into a tailspin and make you worry more than you ever have before.

But as a licensed therapist, I also know that with guidance, it is possible to learn how to mindfully navigate this parenting path with an eye toward managing anxiety, keeping your child safe, and improving your quality of life. Not only is it possible to develop a workable balance between allergy safety and full engagement in life's experiences, but it's also important to do so because letting fear lead your decision-making results in more anxiety and overwhelm—for yourself, your child, and your entire family. I've worked with parents on this very goal, helping them transition from navigating allergy parenting on anxiety autopilot to parenting with mindful intention and developing their "just right" approach to allergy parenting that isn't dictated by fear. In fact, I've also worked through this myself and continue to do so as I enter each new stage of my son's development. Therefore, I wrote this book because I truly believe that it offers parents the evidence-based insights, guidance, and skills needed to help them develop a workable balance between the fear and overwhelm and a good quality of life when parenting a child with allergies.

Here's my own story about receiving my son's food allergy diagnosis—an experience that probably feels familiar.

For my family, that diagnosis came via a phone call while I was walking around a Thomas the Train event. Less than a week before, I had given my three-year-old son his first peanut butter and jelly sandwich. While I loved Reese's peanut butter cups, my husband and I weren't fans of PB&J sandwiches, so we never made them for our kids. We didn't avoid peanut butter, but we also didn't regularly have it in our home. However, since my youngest was getting ready to go to preschool, I figured I should try giving him peanut butter—just in case. I had known kids managing food allergies, and it sounded so incredibly hard . . . and scary. But since we didn't have food allergies in our family, I truly didn't think much about giving him the sandwich.

And then it happened. After a couple of bites, my son stopped eating. Initially, he just sat there. I was around the corner in the laundry room, but my husband was in the kitchen with him. My son sneezed. Then again. And again! Still thinking it was nothing, but also curious why he kept sneezing, I went into the kitchen to see what was happening. That's when I knew something wasn't right. My son was sneezing nonstop and then furiously started rubbing his eyes. Next, the congestion started. It finally hit me—he was having an allergic reaction!

I had no knowledge of allergic reactions or epinephrine (a medication used to reduce or reverse symptoms of allergic reactions), nor did we have epinephrine at home. Instead, the first thing that popped into my head was the movie Hitch. *You know, the one where Will Smith is a dating guru. In the movie, Will Smith's character has an allergic reaction after eating something and visibly swells up. He goes to the store to get an antihistamine, and the reaction eventually resolves.*

So, I pulled a Hitch. *I ran to the medicine cabinet, grabbed the bottle of antihistamine we had, and gave my son a dose. I thought, Phew—he will get better now! Wrong. Minutes later, he started vomiting, and not the "I ate too much candy, and my tummy doesn't feel well" kind of vomiting. It was projectile vomit, and lots of it. Then he started a weird, yawning type of breathing. That's when I really started to worry and called our pediatrician, who confirmed he was having an allergic reaction.*

I honestly don't remember much else from that moment on because I was in full panic mode at that point. Somehow while talking to the pediatrician, my son's symptoms started to resolve, so we were advised to watch him closely and take him to the emergency room if anything changed. Thankfully, his symptoms continued to get better rather than worse, and the allergic reaction eventually stopped.

Even after such a terrifying experience, I was still in denial about the possibility that he had a food allergy, assuming it was just a fluke reaction rather than what my gut knew was likely true. But that all changed a week later. While walking around the Thomas event, I got the phone call sharing the results of my son's blood test. I can look back at pictures from that day and still feel the exact emotions I felt when the doctor said, "Your son is allergic to peanuts and may be allergic to a few tree nuts, too." And just like that, in that moment, I transitioned from being a relaxed parent to one who was constantly on high alert and always searching for threats to my son's safety.

JUST HOW BIG IS THE ALLERGY PARENTING CLUB?

I think it's safe to say that the Allergy Parenting Club wasn't on your list of groups to join when you became a parent. In fact, you probably hoped that you'd never have to join this club because it sounded like a scary one to be part of. However, since you're reading this book, I'm guessing you're already a member, so welcome!

The term *allergy* seems to be casually thrown around, and therefore, is often misunderstood. An *allergy*, which is among the most common chronic conditions worldwide, is a condition involving an abnormal reaction to a normally harmless substance (an allergen), which the immune system interprets as an invader.[1] To protect us when exposed to allergens, the immune system overreacts, which triggers allergic reactions that include symptoms in various systems of the body. Chronic allergic diseases, including food allergy, allergic asthma, eosinophilic esophagitis, allergic rhinitis, and atopic dermatitis, typically impact peoples' day-to-day functioning and often need ongoing management. Some, particularly food allergies and asthma, are even potentially life-threatening. It's also important to note that allergic diseases don't impact only children—they can persist throughout the lifespan or even start in adulthood. Further, despite the emerging treatments for allergic conditions, there are currently no cures—a fact that on its own induces overwhelm and stress in parents.

So, just how big is this Allergy Parenting Club? Pretty big. While precise prevalence data is lacking, statistics from the International Study of Asthma and Allergies in Childhood (ISAAC) suggests that 0.3% to 20.5% of children aged 6 to 14 years old were diagnosed with allergic diseases, with prevalence rates increasing in most parts of the world.[2] Food allergy prevalence rates suggest that almost 8% of kids in the United States (that's 1 in 13 kids),[3] an estimated 500,000 Canadians under 18 years of age,[4] between 6% and 8% of UK-based children up to 3 years old,[5] and around 10% of infants and 4–8% of children in Australia and New Zealand manage food allergies.[6] Asthma, which is the most common chronic disease in children worldwide, is another allergic disease.[7] In the United States, almost 27 million Americans are diagnosed with asthma, 6.1 million of whom are children.[8]. In the United Kingdom, rates of pediatric asthma are among the highest, with 1 in 11 children under 16 years old being diagnosed with asthma.[9] In Canada, approximately 15–25% of children manage asthma, too.[10] These are just the pediatric food allergy and asthma rates of predominantly English-speaking countries. When parents of children managing other allergic diseases and those living in other countries are factored in, the number of members in the Allergy Parenting Club is likely much higher. I hope that all these statistics help you realize that you're truly not alone and that many others are in the allergy parenting trenches with you.

With so many children diagnosed with allergic diseases, you may be wondering about the psychosocial and quality-of-life impacts for these families. In families managing food allergies, 92% of parents say they're always or occasionally fearful for their food-allergic child's safety, with 75% reporting that food allergies cause fear and anxiety for their family.[11] The most common forms of emotional distress experienced by these parents include food allergy-specific anxiety, general anxiety, worry, fear, sadness, and depression.[12] While mothers may feel more empowered to care for their child's food allergies than fathers, they reported more anxiety, stress, and a greater impact on their quality of life than anyone else in the family, including the food-allergic children themselves.[13] What's more, 40% of parents reported experiencing hostility from other parents when trying to accommodate their child's food allergy, and 25% report that food allergy caused strain on their marriage.[14] For families managing asthma, parents are distressed by the uncertainty and fear of continued symptoms and repeated asthma-related hospitalizations, and those families with lower socioeconomic status and exposure to mold within the home had even greater odds of experiencing a lower quality of life.[15] In addition, the burden that these families experience is exacerbated by anxiety, financial hardships, regular use of medications, and simply caring for an asthmatic child who wakes up with asthma-related symptoms at least once per week.[16]

While some parents get to exit the Allergy Parenting Club when their child outgrows their allergy, others remain lifetime members. No matter the length of your involvement, though, it can be helpful to know that there is growing support for allergy families. Over the last decade, the allergic disease landscape has changed a great deal. Compared with raising a child with allergies even five years ago, parents with older children report that there's more information, support, and resources available now. Here are examples of these positive developments:

- Many allergists now utilize individualized approaches to patient care and incorporate psychosocial support as a component.
- Research studies are now exploring a variety of allergy-related quality-of-life topics, including allergy anxiety, mental health, and racial disparities.

- There's a growing number of allergic disease advocacy organizations and support groups (both online and in person).
- There's increased public awareness about allergic diseases and a growing number of allergy-friendly food and consumer brands.
- Schools are more aware of allergic conditions and are gaining a better understanding about the need for health plans and student accommodations.

Finally, while this book focuses primarily on parenting children with food allergies, I truly believe that the key concepts will feel helpful to parents of children managing other allergic conditions, which is why I use the broader term *allergies*. Thus, when the terms *allergy parents* and *allergy parenting* are used throughout this book, they refer to parenting children with any allergic condition since they all have the potential to impact quality of life due to the unpredictability and uncertainty associated with them. Note, though, that these terms are not being used as "labels," but rather are a shorthand way of talking about parenting children with allergic conditions.

HOW THIS BOOK WILL HELP PARENTS OF CHILDREN WITH ALLERGIES

While receiving my son's diagnosis felt hard, learning how to accept and adapt to life with a food allergy felt even more challenging.

After the reality of my son's diagnosis finally sank in, waves of sadness, anger, and disbelief washed over me, making it hard to figure out how to move forward. The constant "what-if" thoughts just wouldn't stop. What if the antihistamine hadn't worked? Will I ever feel ready to let him go to school? What do I do if I feel like he won't ever be safe outside of our home? How will he ever have a normal life now? Did I somehow cause his food allergy?

I surfed these intense emotional waves for months. But then, the therapist part of my mind kicked in and reminded me that I had to get myself back on solid ground. I had to figure out how to live with a diagnosis we never wanted so that I could function well again. More importantly, I had to do all of this for my son's benefit, because if I didn't, he might go through life feeling excessively anxious and fearful, too, and limit himself because of my feelings about his food allergy.

But just when I thought I had the hang of things, the emotional tidal waves came crashing back in with every new "first," knocking me down each time. Just when I was finally starting to feel confident that my son could stay safe while at preschool, it was time for him to transition to kindergarten, where he would be in a new school, with new staff, and where a new routine would be needed. Crash! There came the next wave, which knocked me down again and left me crying uncontrollably on the floor the night before the first day of kindergarten.

That up-and-down pattern seemed to play out in a variety of "first" scenarios: the first sports team he joined (Will his teammates accommodate and respect his allergy?), the first drop-off birthday party (Will he remember to eat the cupcake I provided?), the first time he went to a friend's house for the afternoon (Will he truly eat only approved snacks)? And these "firsts" just kept coming and coming as my son got older.

Maybe you've experienced these intense emotional waves, too. Perhaps you've even felt like you were able to successfully surf them—at least, until the next one came and knocked you back down. Whatever your allergy parenting experience has been so far, there must have been something about this book that made you believe it would be helpful—and it will be, especially if you answer "yes" to any of these questions:

- Do I wrestle with guilt or blame myself for my child's diagnosis?
- Does the fear of my child having an allergic reaction or asthma attack lead to avoiding people, places, or activities, even if they may be safe enough?
- Does my worry about keeping my child safe lead me to feel like I can't ever make a mistake or make me fear that mistakes will always be life or death?
- Am I willing to approach my anxious thoughts differently, so that parenting a child with allergies doesn't feel so overwhelming?
- Have I lost a part of myself due to the stress of parenting a child with allergies?
- Has parenting a child with allergies impacted my marriage or relationship, causing increased tension, stress, or strain?
- Am I exhausted (and even resentful) due to the ongoing need to educate others and advocate for my child's safety and inclusion?
- Would I parent differently if my anxiety and fear didn't have a hold on me or push me around?

Did you answer "yes" to one or more of these questions? By reading my story throughout this chapter, you've probably picked up on the fact that I would have answered "yes" to many of them at that point in my allergy parenting journey, too.

No matter how long you've been a member of the Allergy Parenting Club, this book offers insights that will help you view and approach allergy parenting differently. If you're the parent of a newly diagnosed child, this book will help you form a solid foundation on which to build, with techniques to help you navigate the overwhelm and develop an empowered mindset. If you've been on this allergy parenting journey for a while, you are likely still navigating through developmental transitions that may feel overwhelming, such as your child's entering school or preparing for college, so you'll benefit from this book, too. In addition, not only will parents benefit from this book, but so will entire families.

If you've already read several allergy management books, visited allergy-focused blogs, and are a member of online support groups, you might find yourself wondering, *What is this book going to tell me that I haven't already learned?*

This book isn't a typical allergy book. It's not a "how to" guide for navigating allergy management. It doesn't offer guidance on epinephrine and inhaler use, label-reading, and strategies for avoiding allergic reactions and asthma attacks. After all, I'm not an allergist, so medical guidance is outside of my clinical scope of practice. It's also not a step-by-step guide to parenting a child with allergies. Instead, this book explores topics beyond the medical diagnosis and allergy management basics. It delves into the emotional aspects of allergy management from a parenting perspective. It explores factors that lead to feeling overwhelmed and anxious when parenting a child with allergies and then provides effective strategies to help you manage that overwhelm so that you can parent the way you want to, not the way your anxious mind tells you to. This book will help you navigate the allergy uncertainty in a way that will help you, your allergic child, and your family flourish.

It's also important to note that while I'm sure parents of children managing life-impacting allergies would love to be provided with specific steps for controlling *all* allergy-related thoughts and feelings—an easy button, of sorts—that's not clinical guidance that's possible to offer, and ultimately, it wouldn't prepare parents to deal with the uncertainty and unpredictability that life with allergies (and life in general) presents. In addition, where one approach might work best for you, another might work best for another parent. Just as one learns how to medically manage one's child's allergy, one also has to learn how to manage the thoughts and feelings associated with living with these diagnoses.

WHAT THIS BOOK WILL HELP YOU DO

As I'm sure you already know, allergy diagnoses come with a flurry of thoughts—everything from *this can't be happening* to *I've got this!* These diagnoses also bring with them a variety of uncomfortable emotions and feelings, such as sadness, grief, guilt, overwhelm, and anger. When your child received their diagnosis, you probably quickly pushed those feelings aside by focusing on being the most effective allergy parent ever—one who never makes mistakes, since your mind likely convinced you that all allergy-related mistakes are catastrophic. (We'll explore that unhelpful thought later.) You have also probably tried ignoring the ongoing fear and anxiety and told yourself that if you just try to control everything, your child will be okay. Sure, dealing with anxious thoughts and feelings may be helpful, but who has time for that? After all, if you ignore feelings long enough, they'll eventually just disappear, right?

Wrong. Just like when you're holding your breath under water in the pool for a long period of time, you eventually need to come back to the surface for air. Our uncomfortable thoughts and feelings are no different. They will resurface at some point on this parenting journey, and therefore, dealing with them in real time is useful. It is perfectly normal to experience difficult thoughts and feelings; learning how to cope with them is the key to managing them and not letting them pull you under and drown you.

You see, the mind sometimes becomes an unhelpful friend, one that has a habit of reigniting anxious thoughts and worries when there's change, transition, uncertainty, and unpredictability—all of which are part of the journey of parenting a child with allergies, no matter which allergic condition your child manages. Even so, what if I told you that trying to ignore these uncomfortable thoughts and feelings results in feeling even more anxious and overwhelmed and that being open to your thoughts and feelings will lead you to a life filled with vitality, connection, and meaning even though it includes allergies?

This book is your guide to navigating and managing the anxiety, stress, and overwhelm associated with parenting a child with allergies. Reading it will help you

- explore the beliefs that determine your mindset about living with allergies,

- build awareness of your anxious thoughts, noticing how they act as obstacles to parenting and living the way you want to,
- understand how avoidance isn't always beneficial and sometimes comes at a cost,
- learn how to mindfully notice and respond differently to anxious thoughts that are brought on by the unpredictability of allergies,
- learn how to develop a new relationship with your anxious thoughts so that they don't continue to dictate your parenting decisions,
- learn how to make choices based on what's important to you so that the allergy is just one aspect of your family—not the whole focus,
- develop your "just-right" mindful, balanced approach to living a fully engaged life even with allergies.

THE FOUNDATION FOR THE GUIDANCE IN THIS BOOK

Before we officially jump into this journey together, I think it's important for me to share where the guidance in this book comes from. Sure, I'm a licensed therapist with a masters in family therapy and over 20 years of clinical experience, so I am qualified to write this book. While I do share insights from my own clinical experiences and interactions with hundreds of parents of children with allergies, the content within this book is grounded in allergy research and evidence-based mindfulness and acceptance principles. Specifically, it's aligned with principles from Acceptance and Commitment

Therapy, or ACT (said like the word, not the individual letters). As such, this book isn't going to tell you how to eliminate all anxiety and anxious thoughts, which isn't possible anyway. It doesn't encourage controlling, avoiding, or fixing anxious, painful, or uncomfortable thoughts and feelings, as much as it might feel better to do so. It also won't label feelings as "good" or "bad," because being willing to feel *all* feelings helps us find balance and live a more deeply connected life.

Instead, this book offers insights and skills that will help you show up each day with the willingness to accept and adjust to the reality of parenting a child with allergies, yet still commit to doing what matters most—even in the face of fear, anxiety, and uncertainty. You'll learn how to become more *psychologically flexible*, or willing to experience whatever thoughts and feelings arise in the moment and then make purposeful choices rather than repeating what's not working well. Being psychologically flexible is like having the ability to surf all types of waves in life and, even when thrown off the surfboard, being able to get back on and ride toward what's most important to you. Becoming more psychologically flexible not only benefits you by helping you adapt to life's many changes, but it's also a key component of mental health and well-being in that it helps to decrease stress and anxiety and improve confidence.[17] You'll also learn strategies to help you take a more balanced approach to life with allergies. Referred to as *relaxed readiness*, this approach to allergy management involves finding a workable level of anxiety that helps you balance vigilance and risk-taking, which allows you to live fully while staying prepared to act (when needed) rather than constantly living in fear or, on the contrary, navigating life without any precautions.

HOW THIS BOOK IS STRUCTURED

Chapters 1 and 2 of this book will help you explore your beliefs about parenting a child with allergies and identify potential parenting traps and dynamics contributing to the overwhelm you are feeling. The third chapter looks at developmentally focused allergy parenting goals and various processes to be mindful of in each stage of your child's development. The next three chapters are where you'll learn concepts and skills that will help you more effectively and mindfully navigate the overwhelm and anxiety associated with parenting a child with allergies. Finally, Chapter 7 is where you'll put it all together and map out a more balanced, mindful allergy parenting plan that isn't dictated by anxiety and overwhelm. Here's more of what we will explore throughout the rest of this book:

Chapter 1, "Exploring Unhelpful Allergy Parenting Narratives," delves into common thoughts and feelings parents experience after their child receives an allergy diagnosis, which often give way to unhelpful narratives that impact their mindset about living with allergies and allergy parenting expectations.

Chapter 2, "Recognizing Common Allergy Parenting Traps" outlines six common allergy parenting traps that can push parents farther away from a balanced, mindful approach to life with allergies, including needing certainty, engaging in over-avoidance and over-functioning, making comparisons, drowning in burnout, and battling with resentment.

Chapter 3, "Setting Developmentally Focused Allergy Parenting Goals," explores the "relaxed readiness" approach to life with allergies and presents a mindful parenting framework to help you set allergy parenting goals that are focused on balancing your child's development, your own parenting development, and the development of allergy management skills throughout each age and stage.

Chapter 4, "Responding Differently to Anxious Thoughts," offers a primer on anxiety, explores unhelpful approaches for managing anxious thoughts, and provides you with ACT-aligned strategies for responding to anxious thoughts more mindfully so that you can develop a new relationship with your allergy anxiety.

Chapter 5, "Focusing on All That Matters—Not Just Allergy Safety," introduces the concept of values and explores how values help you develop the willingness to keep moving towards all that's important (not just allergy safety) even when there are obstacles in the way, including allergy anxiety, overwhelm, and fear.

Chapter 6, "Developing Flexible Perspectives on Allergy Parenting," focuses on shifting your perspective from one that's focused primarily on fear and overwhelm to one that allows you to consider more flexible outcomes, as well as the benefits of practicing self-compassion as an allergy parent.

Chapter 7, "Putting Your Balanced, Mindful Allergy Parenting Plan into Action," brings together everything you've learned throughout the book so that you can begin mapping out your values-aligned parenting plan to help you navigate allergy parenting with acceptance, mindfulness, and balance.

While not required, I highly recommend having a notebook or journal to use while reading this book. Don't worry—I'm not going to ask you to spend time each night writing a Dear Diary entry in it. The journal will be where you answer exploratory questions and take additional notes that will help you reflect on what you're reading. Plus, keeping this journal will allow you to visually see the growth you've made over time.

I'll address one last thought you might have after reading this far: *I know I'm anxious about allergies, but shouldn't I be? Won't my anxiety help me keep my child from getting very sick or even worse, dying?*

While your mind wants you to believe that anxiety is what will keep your child safe, it's not that simple. This book will teach you how to discern between useful and problematic anxiety and how to engage with your allergy-related thoughts in a way that doesn't make every choice feel like a life-or-death debate.

Are you wondering how I made the transition from letting the overwhelm of parenting a child with allergies derail me to now writing a therapeutic book for allergy parents? Here's the rest of my story about my entrance into the Allergy Parenting Club, and the very moment I decided it was time to become the parent I wanted to be rather than the one my allergy anxiety was pushing me to become.

Somewhere along the way, my goal of just getting through each day as an allergy parent became a goal to teach my son that he could be resilient with a food allergy, even at a young age. I couldn't imagine our family living in fear our whole lives! But I knew that if I wanted my son to learn how to be resilient, it was up to me to pave the way first. While living with a food allergy was scary, I needed to teach myself, and then my son, how to find a workable balance between seeking safety (to avoid reactions) and enjoying life's experiences. It was my job as the parent to help us both work toward accepting, adjusting, and adapting to this new reality.

I started by creating my own emotional survival raft built on acceptance and allergy knowledge, which kept me from emotionally drowning. Then I focused on building new allergy parenting narratives—ones that reminded me that even with this diagnosis and my fears, my son could still have a safe and wonderfully fun life. I often wondered if I would be able to continue navigating the intense emotional battle that was taking place in my mind each day. But if it meant helping my son learn how to live the best life he could even with a food allergy, then without a doubt—I would find a way through it.

And so will you!

While this may be the end of the introduction, it's just the beginning—the beginning of a new, more mindful and balanced approach to life with allergies for you and your whole family. It's time to turn off anxiety autopilot and be the parent (and family) you want to be!

CHAPTER 1

Exploring Unhelpful Allergy Parenting Narratives

In preparation for this book, I asked hundreds of parents of children with food allergies to answer the following question: "When my child was diagnosed with a food allergy, I felt ________ and thought ____________." Below is a handful of their responses illustrating just how common it is to feel overwhelmed by an allergy diagnosis:

- I felt overwhelmed and wondered how I would protect her.
- I felt overwhelmed and thought I had to do everything right.
- I felt surprised and thought it was my fault.
- I felt responsible and thought, "How do I fix this?"
- I felt uneducated and thought I was alone.
- I felt anger and grief over losing my normal life.
- I felt scared and thought I could lose my only child to accidental microscopic exposure to her allergen.
- I felt disbelief and thought this isn't happening to us—we don't have food allergies in our family!
- I felt devastated and thought that she would never have a normal childhood as she would be excluded from most

events at school, among her peers, and that she couldn't be safe without me. I mourned for weeks.

- I felt surprised, and I thought it would be easier. I didn't understand the amount of stress and fear we were about to face for years.
- I felt relieved to know why my baby had been so unwell and uncomfortable since birth, albeit overwhelmed and thought at least we can start moving forward.

One of the parents who responded to this question messaged me privately to expand on her answer. She had been an allergy parent for a decade but shared how her son's dairy allergy initially felt impossible to manage because so many foods included dairy. The terrifying news stories about food allergy-related fatalities had scared her so much that she found herself believing that the world wasn't safe for her son. In response, she determined that the only way to maintain safety was to keep him away from others and even held him back from attending preschool. She shared that while doing this helped her feel less overwhelmed, she began noticing that keeping her son away from others not only negatively affected his social skills, but also led him to believe that the world wasn't safe for him—which made her feel incredibly sad. Even though she was able to reflect on this in hindsight, she emphasized how her initial allergy-related beliefs had been unhelpful and affected her family's ability to accept her son's diagnosis and adjust to life with a food allergy.

MAKING SENSE OF THE OVERWHELM

As you reflect on your child's diagnosis experience, can you relate to any (or all) of these parent responses?

Since many children get diagnosed with allergic diseases during infancy and toddlerhood, the diagnosis adds an extra layer of stress when life already feels stressful. So it's understandable to feel overwhelmed by an allergy diagnosis, especially because there's a lot of information to digest and many lifestyle changes to make once the initial shock wears off.

When an experience feels overwhelming, our mind is desperate to make sense of the chaos to avoid feeling intense pain. What helps us make sense of it is language, which allows us to describe, evaluate, and analyze our experiences.[1] We do this by creating internal narratives, or stories we tell ourselves about who we are, the world around us, and how we function in it. Simply stated, internal narratives are our mind's way of putting complex beliefs, feelings, and situations into a context we can understand so that we can more effectively navigate something that feels difficult.

In his book *Families, Illness, and Disability*, psychiatrist John Rolland states that the challenges of living with a chronic health condition affect the entire family system, not just the person who was diagnosed. To create order out of chaos and fear, the family develops their core beliefs about the diagnosis and constructs a narrative that answers questions such as *Why me? Why us? Why now?* and *What can we do?*[2] Rolland also emphasizes that belief systems and narratives significantly impact how families navigate health conditions since they serve as maps that shape how families interpret events, as well as guide the decisions they make and the actions they take in managing the condition.

For many families, these initial allergy beliefs and narratives typically feel unhelpful and discouraging: *This is too overwhelming for us to manage*. For others, their initial allergy beliefs and narratives feel helpful and empowering: *We can do this even though it feels overwhelming.* This is especially the case if their child experienced ongoing unknown reactions or health issues without an identified cause, which can be the case for children with asthma or food protein-induced enterocolitis (FPIES). When children receive such a diagnosis, parents might feel like they've found the missing piece to a confusing puzzle and had their parental intuition that something wasn't right validated.

Whatever your initial allergy narrative, one main benefit of developing an awareness of it is that it helps you assess whether it is hindering or helping your adjustment—that is, is it helping or not helping you to learn how to live a full life even with allergies? In addition, as you'll hear repeatedly throughout this book, there's value in being willing to feel all emotions and observe all thoughts, and in future chapters, you'll learn how to relate to uncomfortable emotions and thoughts in healthier ways. But then, since we're quick to push pain away, you likely didn't reflect on the initial narratives you created when your child was diagnosed—especially the unhelpful ones that affected your ability to accept and adjust to the diagnosis, which may still be influencing you now. Yet reflecting on these narratives not only helps you assess if and how you have adjusted to life with allergies, but also allows you to gain perspective on how far you've come as an allergy parent and determine what helps you lead your family toward living the life you want even with your child's diagnosis.

COMMON ALLERGY PARENTING NARRATIVES AFTER DIAGNOSIS

Most of the previous parent responses fit into four common unhelpful allergy parenting narratives—ones that many of the hundreds of parents I've interacted with have engaged with after their child was diagnosed. While these unhelpful narratives are most common at diagnosis and during the adjustment to living with allergies, they can (and often do) persist or resurface after specific events, especially after allergic reactions or asthma attacks and at developmental transitions in your child's life. When you continue to let these unhelpful narratives guide you after the initial adjustment to the diagnosis, it's easy to stay in struggle mode with your emotions and thoughts, which leads you farther away from accepting your new normal.

Below are those four common unhelpful allergy parenting narratives. As you read through them, consider which ones might have been present at the time of your child's diagnosis and whether they might still be impacting how you parent today. The information you'll learn throughout this book will help you meet the underlying emotions and thoughts associated with these narratives more flexibly so that you can learn how to parent based on your goals rather than fear and overwhelm.

The *Not What I Expected* Narrative

Rachel had been dreaming of being a parent for years, so when she learned she was pregnant, she could hardly contain her joy. She was excited for every first—first words, first steps, and the first birthday party with a separate smash cake for her child to tear into.

When Rachel's daughter was six months old, she was diagnosed with a dairy allergy after experiencing anaphylaxis while eating yogurt. She was also diagnosed with a peanut allergy at around eight months old, which increased the anxiety Rachel was already experiencing about keeping her daughter safe. Now managing two food allergies, Rachel found herself incredibly sad instead of excited as she prepared for her daughter's first birthday. Her mind was constantly ruminating about how reality wasn't lining up with her expectations for parenthood. She had even convinced herself that the vision she had for her daughter's birthday was ruined because her daughter couldn't eat a traditional birthday cake. In fact, she felt sure that her daughter would never have a normal birthday celebration.

At her daughter's allergy appointment one week before her first birthday, Rachel shared these thoughts with the allergist, who reassured her that experiencing grief and noticing loss are normal when adjusting to life with allergies. The doctor also shared that it's not uncommon for parents to notice grief popping up again with each new age and stage their child goes through. To help Rachel reimagine her daughter's first birthday party with a focus on safety *and* fun, the allergist provided Rachel with a list of allergy-friendly brands that sold dairy-free and peanut-free cake mixes. Suddenly, Rachel reconnected with excitement again as she realized that the vision she had for her daughter's birthday was possible, just with a different, safe cake!

Rachel's story is a great example of the *Not What I Expected* narrative. This narrative is rooted primarily in grief and loss since an allergy diagnosis signals drastic changes, as well as a departure from normalcy and what you had envisioned for your child's life. In addition to grief, the most common feelings associated with this narrative are sadness, numbness, defeat, pain, and devastation. These emotions give way to beliefs such as *life will never be the same*; *this condition will ruin my child's life*; and *I don't know how to find joy now that my child has an allergy.*

Grief is a normal emotional response that arises as you move through the process of accepting and adjusting to loss, such as the loss of normalcy. When parenting a child diagnosed with allergies, grieving often feels complex as you're focused on the current adjustments while also fearing future grief-inducing experiences. Like anticipatory anxiety, which causes our mind to focus on worries about what's to come, anticipatory grief hits when you think about the threat and uncertainty the allergy imposes on your child's future. In response to those perceived threats, the mind likes to engage with rigid, rule-like thoughts that include terms like *always* and *never*, such as Rachel's thought *my child will never have a normal birthday celebration.* Unfortunately, these beliefs can lead you to engage in unhelpful actions such as setting unrealistic rules about how to keep your child safe (in service of protecting yourself from more grief) and hyper-focusing on how you wish things would be different, which keeps you feeling stuck in sadness and pain and less willing to take actions focused on moving forward. Grief can also show up when your expectations for parenthood don't line up with the reality you're experiencing. So, how should you manage this grief and loss?

You may be familiar with one of the most well-known theories about loss called the Five Stages of Grief developed by psychiatrist Elisabeth Kubler-Ross. The stages of grief are denial (*this can't be happening to us*), anger (*why is this happening to us?*), bargaining (*I will do anything to change this*), depression (*how will life ever be good again?*), and acceptance (*it's going to be okay—we can do this*).[3] Kubler-Ross's long-time collaborator, David Kessler, also developed a sixth stage known as *finding meaning*.[4] While these stages illustrate that addressing grief is a process, it's not a linear process, and therefore, we can (and often do) move back and forth through these stages at any point in time. In fact, grief doesn't go away—and we don't need it to go away to move forward after a painful experience.

Another theory about loss, and the one I find most useful in helping allergy parents accept and adapt to life with allergies, is psychologist Lois Tonkin's model of Growing Around Grief. This theory states that painful feelings may always be present, but through the pursuit of new experiences, we can reconnect with joy even in the presence of grief.[5] To help visualize this, imagine a jar with a ball inside of it. The ball represents grief, and the jar represents life. Even though we might assume that the ball (grief) shrinks over time, it doesn't—it stays the same size. Instead, the jar (life) gets bigger over time so that grief doesn't monopolize all the space, which then allows space for joyful feelings and experiences, too.

How reassuring is it to read that we don't have to eliminate pain to reconnect with happiness? Every time I share this with a parent, I see a physical release of tension as they begin to reimagine a path forward that allows for both loss and joy. I hope you're feeling a sense of relief as you read this, too. And so when grief resurfaces again on this allergy parenting journey—and it will—remember that your goal is to move forward and grow around the pain and that both time and allergy parenting experiences will help you do so.

The *This Can't Be Happening* Narrative

Matt's son had been diagnosed with asthma and multiple food allergies. As someone who prided himself on his ability to find solutions to challenges in life, realizing that his son's diagnoses couldn't be "fixed" left him feeling helpless as a parent. He struggled to accept that he couldn't make these allergic diseases go away and felt like he wouldn't be able to keep his son safe from all the possible threats outside of the home. His belief that he couldn't make things better for his son often brought about a variety of emotions, including anger, frustration, and jealousy when thinking about families who didn't manage allergies. This gave way to racing thoughts and rumination about how unfair it felt that his child was managing multiple diagnoses.

The emotional overwhelm from all of this eventually led him to start disengaging from daily allergy and asthma management tasks. He was willing to help his partner with other parenting and household tasks, but to try and shield himself from feeling helpless, he avoided talking about and helping manage the asthma and food allergies. Unfortunately, this created conflict within his marriage and while there was temporary relief from his thoughts, this approach ultimately made him feel worse in the long term.

Matt's story is an example of the *This Can't Be Happening* narrative, which makes you feel like you're living through one of your worst nightmares—one where you don't wake up and realize it was a dream. The primary feelings associated with this narrative include anger, frustration, denial, disbelief, shock, and even jealousy of others who don't manage allergies. While these are normal and expected emotional responses to an allergy diagnosis, especially if the experiences leading up to it were traumatic, if you are dominated by this narrative beyond the adjustment period, you'll find it harder to accept and adapt to life with the allergy. This narrative often gives way to thoughts such as, *Why is this happening to my child and not others?*; *I don't want this to be our reality*; and *This is unfair.*

Thanks to our prehistoric ancestors who were always on high alert to stay safe, our minds are hard-wired with a survival instinct that encourages us to avoid uncomfortable situations in case they're dangerous. Unfortunately, this instinct tends to work overtime, as it also encourages us to avoid and disconnect from uncomfortable thoughts and feelings. And if we do encounter them, we often take actions aimed at getting rid of them as quickly as possible, typically without much consideration for how these actions affect us in the long term.

The unwillingness to remain in contact with uncomfortable internal experiences (thoughts, feelings, and memories) by actively trying to escape, avoid, change, or eliminate them is called *experiential avoidance*.[6] When you're struggling to come to terms with your child's diagnosis, you might find yourself engaging in experiential avoidance by becoming preoccupied by wishful thoughts that your child's allergy will suddenly go away. Or perhaps you keep telling yourself to stop feeling angry and just deal with it. Maybe you even engage in more obvious avoidance behaviors such as scrolling through social media for hours or drinking just to keep your distance from the discomfort you experience from your thoughts and feelings.

While avoiding and escaping our internal experiences makes us believe we're minimizing suffering and pain, the relief we feel is temporary. Why? Because it's impossible to avoid our thoughts and feelings forever, and trying to do so leads only to experiencing more internal struggles. Additionally, feeling pain is part of the human experience. As such, it's normal for allergy parents to notice feelings such as anger, disbelief, and shock when their child is diagnosed—and trying to disconnect from these emotions isn't going to make them go away. Your child's diagnosis also isn't likely to go away, which means that at some point, you're going to have to face the internal discomforts associated with parenting a child with allergies.

But what do I mean when I say that you'll need to face the discomfort? I mean being willing to allow *all* thoughts and feelings about your child's allergy (even uncomfortable ones like fear, anxiety, sadness, and anger) and to be present without trying to control or resist them—to simply give them space to exist. A core process of Acceptance and Commitment Therapy (ACT) is *acceptance*, or having the willingness to be open to all thoughts and feelings. This *acceptance* helps us become more *psychologically flexible*, or better able to accept and adapt to what life presents us.[7] We will delve much deeper into acceptance and experiential avoidance in future chapters. For now, I simply want you to be mindful of the fact that being willing to experience discomfort rather than avoiding it is a crucial component of learning how to navigate allergy parenting the way you want to rather than the way fear dictates.

The *It's My Fault* Narrative

When Devika's son was seven months old, he developed a few hives around his mouth after eating eggs. Figuring it was just a bit of irritation, Devika gave him some eggs again, only this time, he developed hives all over his body and began vomiting. After calling the pediatrician, they went to his office the next day, where her son received an egg allergy diagnosis and a referral to follow up with a board-certified allergist for more guidance. As she prepared for the allergist appointment, Devika was overcome with regret and self-blame as her mind ruminated over every detail. She began listing all the ways in which she was sure her son's diagnosis was her fault: she ate eggs daily while pregnant, she underwent a C-section to deliver him, she didn't breastfeed him, and her judgment was poor since she fed him eggs even after he developed hives. The guilt she began carrying felt physically heavy.

When they met with the allergist, she told him that she didn't feel she could trust that her own decisions would keep her son safe given she felt that his diagnosis was her fault. The allergist reassured her that her son's egg allergy wasn't her fault and shared data debunking common food allergy causation myths. He also informed her that current feeding guidelines encourage parents to introduce common allergens early and often but noted that there was no certainty that introducing her son to eggs earlier would have prevented his allergy. After hearing all of this, the relief immediately washed over Devika. The information the allergist shared allowed her to stop blaming herself, regain trust in her parenting capabilities, and refocus her energy on learning how to keep her son healthy and safe.

Devika's story is a good example of the *It's My Fault* narrative, also known as the "blame game." Let's face it—it's easier to blame yourself for your child's allergy than sit with unanswered questions and uncertainty about the future, right? The most common feelings associated with this narrative are sadness, guilt, self-blame, self-doubt, regret, and even shame. This narrative is grounded in beliefs including *my child was diagnosed with an allergy because of something I did or didn't do*; *the reaction was my fault*; and *I lack good enough judgment to keep my child safe*.

All too often, parents blame themselves for their child's allergy. Because the mind is a threat-seeking machine, it wants to locate and decrease all threats while increasing safety and predictability. Our mind tells us that there *must* be answers to explain why the allergy developed, so we start looking for answers everywhere—even if there aren't answers to find or the answers we find are incorrect. Even without evidence supporting the notion that parents' actions cause children's allergies, self-blame provides a sense of certainty. It's *an* answer even if it's not the *correct* answer.

Just as Devika's son's allergist told her, the good news is that current research acts as an antidote to allergy parent self-blame. In *The End of Food Allergy*, doctor Kari Nadeau shares that "for all that we don't know about food allergy, we have enough evidence to assuage the blame."[8] Nadeau offers more reassurance in her book by addressing common guilt-producing food allergy causation themes: maternal diet during pregnancy and breastfeeding (no clear evidence that diet causes food allergies, so moms are encouraged to focus on nutrition and diversification of foods); breastfeeding versus formula feeding (no clear evidence that either leads to or prevents food allergies); and delivering via cesarean section (no conclusive evidence linking the two). Genetics is another common source of self-blame, but understanding the role genes play in the development of allergic diseases is complex. While there's no such thing as food allergy or asthma genes, a variety of allergic disease studies have uncovered data to suggest that there is a hereditary element to these diagnoses. With that said, much more research is still needed in this area. Given the complexity of genetics, and since medical guidance is outside of my scope of practice as a mental health practitioner, I encourage you to discuss any genetic concerns (and self-blame tendencies) with your allergist so they can provide you with current data in the context of your child's specific diagnosis and your family history.

Speaking of conversations with allergists—your child's allergy care team is an important resource as you try to make sense of the allergy. Don't be afraid to tell them if you're experiencing self-blame, especially if it's hindering your ability to adjust to life with allergies, as they'll be able to provide you with information that will help you drop the struggle with guilt. You will not be the first or the last family to express emotions surrounding your child's diagnosis, and most allergists have seen the vast variety of responses and can be helpful in assuaging some of your concerns. But if you don't feel that your child's allergist is well-versed in the current research and isn't using current best practices to guide patient care, then locate a board-certified allergist who does. Your ability to alter this narrative (and many others) is directly influenced by your trust (or lack thereof) in your allergist's guidance. You can locate a board-certified allergist using the Allergist Finder tool on the websites of national allergy and immunology professional networks such as the American Academy of Allergy, Asthma & Immunology and the American College of Allergy, Asthma & Immunology (or the equivalent in your country). Visit the resource section at the back of this book for more guidance.

The *I Can't Do This* Narrative

Ann's daughter had been diagnosed with multiple food allergies around six months old. Initially, Ann felt she could manage the allergies well, but when her daughter started walking and exploring the world, Ann no longer felt she could keep her daughter safe. She wanted to be an allergy parent who approached life with more balance—able to pursue fun experiences and let her daughter do age-appropriate things while also feeling confident that she could handle any uncertainty or reactions that arose. Unfortunately, she believed that she didn't function well under pressure because in past anxiety-inducing experiences, she tended to freeze and was unable to take quick action. As in the cliché "You can't teach an old dog new tricks," Ann believed that she would never be able to learn how to confidently respond to allergic reactions and didn't even want to try. She had resigned herself to being someone who wouldn't take her daughter anywhere unless someone else accompanied them.

Ann's story is an example of the *I Can't Do This* narrative, which is typically based on the belief that you are incapable of managing your child's allergy or that you don't have the necessary skills to do so. The most common emotions associated with this narrative are anxiety, fear, overwhelm, insecurity, and confusion. This narrative is often triggered by thoughts such as *I'm not capable of managing allergies well*; *I need to control everything to keep my child healthy and safe*; and *the world is too unsafe for children with allergies.*

It's understandable to feel as though you're not well equipped to manage your child's allergy, especially after they've just been diagnosed or if you're new to allergic diseases. However, the *I Can't Do This* narrative goes beyond that thought. It's a mindset that makes you believe that you aren't capable of being a good allergy parent and that even with guidance from the allergist, you don't think you ever will be.

Mindset is a concept popularized by psychologist Carol Dweck's research on implicit beliefs, which tells us that how you view yourself directly impacts how you navigate life.[9] The metaphor I use to describe mindset involves eye-glasses:

Your view of yourself (and others) is affected by which pair of glasses you're wearing. More specifically, people wear either fixed mindset glasses or growth mindset glasses. In her book *Mindset: The New Psychology of Success*, Dweck explains that a *fixed mindset* means that you believe that the qualities you possess are permanent and can't be changed (e.g., *I am not smart*), whereas a *growth mindset* is based on the belief that your qualities can be enhanced through efforts to learn, practice, and grow (e.g., *I have the ability to learn*).[10]

One's mindset also has a direct impact on health perceptions or views about health and illness and affects how one chooses to manage health conditions. In a study exploring the health mindset and behaviors of teens managing type 1 diabetes, researchers found that a growth mindset was associated with greater frequency of glucose monitoring.[11] As an allergy parent, your mindset directly impacts your thoughts about what living with an allergy means for your child, as well as the actions you take to keep your child healthy and safe. A fixed mindset tends to give way to increased psychological stress and unhelpful thoughts that fuel anxiety rather than leading you to engage in purposeful actions that help you effectively manage the allergy. For instance, your mind convinces you that no matter how much you practice with self-administered epinephrine device trainers, it won't make you more capable of responding to emergencies effectively. As such, you're more likely to avoid situations that you perceive to be unsafe even if they're safe enough for your child, which makes living with an allergy feel harder than it should.

By contrast, a growth mindset helps you cultivate resilience and persistence in the face of challenges, as it allows you to envision yourself getting through tough situations such as allergic reactions. It helps you interpret allergy-related challenges as speedbumps rather than roadblocks, encouraging you to be solution-focused and to build skills that help you navigate challenges rather than assume things are impossible. With a growth mindset, you can remind yourself that even though you may not feel confident in new situations *yet*, with time and practice, you will.

In Ann's story, what she hadn't considered is that even though she believed she was incapable of handling emergencies effectively, she could learn how to do so. Through information-gathering and practice, Ann could cultivate the skills that would enable her to calmly address an allergic reaction, which would increase her confidence in her allergy parenting capabilities and empower her to go on solo excursions with her daughter.

Thanks to neuroplasticity, or the process that allows the brain to change through exposure to information, mindful awareness of perceptions, and adjustment of internal self-talk, mindsets can change.[12] In addition, you may notice that it feels easier to engage with a growth mindset in some situations rather than others. With time, more allergy parenting experiences, and by using the skills which you'll gain from this book, you can learn how to walk through this journey with a growth mindset even when things feel overwhelming. All you need is the willingness and commitment to learn how. The first step is becoming aware of the thoughts, beliefs, and internal narratives you're experiencing about your child's allergy, which this chapter is helping you do. Use the examples in Table 1.1 to help you continue exploring whether your allergy-related mindset is fixed or growth-focused.

Table 1.1 Growth Mindset and Fixed Mindset About Allergies

Growth Mindset	Fixed Mindset
• It's okay to have all kinds of thoughts and feelings about my child's allergy.	• If I feel anxious about my child's allergy, it means I'm not a good allergy parent.
• If my child has an allergic reaction, I will follow our emergency action plan.	• If my child has an allergic reaction, I won't be brave enough to use epinephrine.
• Navigating new situations feels challenging but helps me grow as an allergy parent.	• I'm not capable of keeping my child safe in new situations, so I will avoid them.
• We can learn how to safely eat out, travel, and attend holiday gatherings with practice.	• Doing things safely outside of the home feels too hard, so we shouldn't even try.

BE OPEN TO NEW PERSPECTIVES AND NARRATIVES

While most of these unhelpful allergy parenting narratives feel discouraging, the good news is that your beliefs and narratives will change on this journey (and may already have). With time and experience, and as your family develops their allergy management skills, you'll be able to engage in different perspectives that will help you adjust your allergy parenting narratives to be empowering rather than discouraging. It's like the different perspectives you might have before and after hiking up a mountain. As you're standing at the base of the mountain gearing up for your hike, it makes sense to feel anxious and wonder, *Can I really do this?* Hiking up a mountain is a challenging task, especially if you haven't had much training. But the farther you get into your hike and the closer you get to the top, the more capable and confident you feel because you can see how far you've come, which helps you to keep going. By the time you reach the bottom again, you're able to look at the hike from a new perspective—one that allows you to adjust your narratives about hiking and your own capabilities as a hiker.

Consider your child's allergic diagnosis as the mountain you're hiking up. The only way to get to the top is to take it one step at a time. Just as no hiker gets from the base of the mountain to the top in one giant leap, you won't master all the ins and outs of allergy parenting all at once either. Take this allergy parenting hike one step at a time and focus on ensuring you have the right equipment and support, which will help you make progress and allow your perspectives to shift, too.

The parent responses shared at the beginning of the chapter represent the perspectives at the start of the allergy parenting hike when you're questioning everything. To gather allergy parenting perspectives shaped by time and experience, I asked this follow-up question: "If my current self could give my former self any advice at the time of my child's diagnosis, that advice would be ________." Here's what a handful of parents had to say as they got farther up the mountain, which hopefully helps you envision a more manageable future with allergies:

- It will get easier.
- Take deep breaths—you can do this!
- You will find a new normal.
- Everything is going to be okay!
- Establish a support group and have faith.
- You will learn how to keep your baby safe.
- Surround yourself with the people who support you the most.

- Keep your positive mindset, and don't let all the "what-if" scenarios bog you down.
- Don't focus on the future and what you can't control; focus on now and small daily wins.
- Your child will be okay; you will find ways to ensure they will live life to the fullest and not miss out.

LET VALUES GUIDE YOUR FAMILY'S ALLERGY BELIEFS AND NARRATIVES

In *Families, Illness, and Disability*, Rolland also mentions that although individual family members may hold different beliefs about living with a diagnosis, the beliefs and values held by the family unit have an incredible influence on how they cope and move forward.[13] In ACT, *values* refer to the qualities we embody—ones that give our lives meaning as we navigate the world. Unlike goals, which are tasks we aim to accomplish or achieve, values function like a compass, guiding our actions and choices in life. They help us behave in ways that align with who we want to be and what we want to stand for, and they also help us understand what matters most in our lives and in our relationships. Examples of values include, but certainly aren't limited to, courage, curiosity, gratitude, honesty, humor, kindness, integrity, mindfulness, persistence, safety, and supportiveness.

We'll dive much deeper into values in Chapter 5, so this section is simply planting the values seed. The values that guide your family will help you develop allergy-related beliefs and narratives that feel empowering rather than discouraging. They'll also help you ensure that you're taking actions in service of what matters to your family in addition to protecting your child. Safety is obviously a key value for allergy families and one you'll always prioritize, so as you continue reading this book, I recommend considering other values on which to focus. For example, maybe bravery is a value that you feel is important to engage with as your family encounters the challenges of living with allergies. Perhaps gratitude is something you'd like your family to practice regularly to help you stay connected to joy. Or maybe persistence is needed to keep you moving forward even when anxiety and grief are present.

In my family, flexibility is one of many values that are important because being flexible is how I want my kids to approach life. When my youngest was diagnosed with his peanut allergy, my first instinct was to become very controlling to keep him safe. I developed very rigid, inflexible routines that I always enforced. For example, I didn't allow food into the house unless I called the manufacturer to confirm its safety first. We also stopped going out anywhere that had food, including restaurants, movie theaters, play places, and others' houses. Even though I felt I was doing a good job keeping my youngest safe, I quickly realized that the rigid rules and routines were taking a toll on me and my whole family. I was tired from being on the phone each day, which also kept me from being able to spend time with my kids. We were also missing out on fun experiences with friends and family, which left us feeling disconnected from others. I had replaced flexibility with rigidity, and because of this, our family's allergy narrative became *the world is not a safe place when you have allergies.* Life felt very hard and not the least bit enjoyable.

I had a literal Oprah a-ha moment when I realized that by living in such a rigid, rule-governed way, I was abandoning our deeply important family value of flexibility. I worked with my own therapist to reconnect with other values I had cast aside when I was concerned only with safety, which helped me learn how to focus on (and prioritize) more than one value at a time. While it didn't happen overnight, our family learned how to live flexibly *and* safely with allergies. We developed more workable ways of establishing which foods were safe, learned how to assess a restaurant's safety profile, and even began taking vacations via air travel again.

Just as every child's allergy profile is unique, each family's allergy journey will be unique, too. Being mindful of the allergy parenting beliefs and narratives you started this journey with will not only help you reflect on your adjustment to the diagnosis but will also help your family determine when you need to lean into your values to develop new narratives that allow your family to live safely *and* fully.

TAKEAWAYS

- It's normal to feel a wide array of emotions when your child is diagnosed with an allergic disease and to initially feel overwhelmed.
- To make sense of the overwhelm, families often develop beliefs and narratives that guide them, some of which are unhelpful.
- Being aware of your allergy beliefs and narratives is important, as they impact your ability to adjust to life with allergies.

- Remember that with time and experience, your allergy beliefs, narratives, and perspectives will likely change—you won't always feel the same as you do in this current moment.

Think About and Do

- Think about the allergy beliefs and narratives that were guiding you when your child was diagnosed and the ones guiding you now. Are they currently the same or different?
- Which of your beliefs and narratives empower you to make parenting decisions based on what's important to your family? Which beliefs and narratives push you to make decisions in response to fear and other intense emotions?
- Begin creating your own list of allergy-related growth mindset-focused statements to help you navigate the overwhelm. As you continue reading, you'll likely add more to this list!

CHAPTER 2

Recognizing Common Allergy Parenting Traps

There's no doubt that parenting a child with allergies is hard. You have to keep your child safe, but not sheltered. You're meant to be cautious, but not overly worried about their health. You're tasked with teaching your child how to manage their allergy while not making them feel anxious about having it. You must teach your child how to embrace their differences, while also helping them navigate feeling left out in some situations.

What makes allergy parenting even harder is getting caught in *allergy parenting traps*–behavioral patterns that seem helpful in the short term but create more struggle in the long term. What's more, parents aren't always aware that they're stuck in one or more of these traps. Often, parents believe they're taking actions that are in service of their child's safety, but the way in which they pursue that goal leads them into these traps. Once in them, it's hard for parents to get out because they've convinced themselves that their actions are what's keeping their child healthy and safe. Unfortunately, this comes at the entire family's expense since staying stuck in these traps typically impacts child development, parental development (even beyond just allergy parenting), familial and marital relationships, self-care, and daily functioning.

The six allergy parenting traps described in this chapter were developed after observing common themes that make it harder for parents to accept and adapt to life with allergies. The strategies that are aligned with Acceptance and Commitment Therapy (ACT), presented in future chapters, will further help you climb out of these traps, so for now, just familiarize yourself with them, consider which traps you may have been or are currently stuck in, and use the exit tips to begin changing unhelpful actions and patterns. As you read through this chapter, you might find yourself thinking, *I have to keep taking these actions to keep my child healthy and safe*. If you are, remind yourself that the goal of allergy parenting is to maintain your child's health and safety while also fully engaging in day-to-day life, which these traps often keep you, your child, and your family from doing.

THE COMPARISON TRAP

Ever find yourself spending hours online to see how everyone else manages their child's allergic condition? Information-gathering to reassure yourself that you're the best allergy parent you can be is at the core of the Comparison Trap. Often, these comparisons happen while surfing through posts on social media and online allergy groups.

One parent recently told me, "Because I'm new to allergy parenting, when I notice I'm feeling anxious and uncertain about how to keep my son safe outside of our home, I visit online allergy groups to learn from others who are probably better allergy parents than me because they're more experienced." She didn't feel confident yet as an allergy parent and believed that learning from others would help her realize that she was doing a good job. She went on to say, "Sometimes I feel better after reading how others safely approach things such as birthday parties and playdates, but other times, because there are so many ways people handle social situations, I walk away convinced I'm not doing a good enough job and am even more confused. Then I try to find information via Google to sort out the confusion, but I eventually give up because my head is spinning." What this parent noticed was that going online to seek reassurance led to navigating an abundance of information, some of which was conflicting and made her question her family's allergy management strategies even more.

Many allergy parents have told me that visiting online allergy groups leads to experiencing an internal tug-of-war between relief and anxiety, as there are both benefits and costs of engaging in these groups. On one hand, finding support, building community, and learning that you're not alone in your experiences are all valuable, especially if your child is newly diagnosed. On the other hand, having access to such specific details about everyone's day-to-day allergy management can result in your feeling overwhelmed and questioning your allergy management approaches even more. For example, two common topics food allergy parents tend to compare are whether to call food manufacturers to learn about allergen protocols and whether to allow their child to eat foods with precautionary labels such as "made in a facility with allergens." Should you be calling every manufacturer? Are you a bad allergy parent if you don't? What if you feel comfortable giving your child foods that may contain their allergen even though many others don't? Questions such as these can easily give way to the Comparison Trap, but you should address these kinds of concerns with your allergist rather than making decisions based on others' experiences.

It's also important to pay attention to what kind of allergy information you're engaging with online. *Evidence-based information*, which is derived from available research and shared by qualified professionals, is different from lived experience–based information, which consists of personal experiences and is often what's shared in online allergy groups. Both types of information are valuable for different reasons, but it's important to consider what type of information is best when exploring allergy-related uncertainties. *Lived experience–based information* helps you gain different perspectives on allergy parenting, which may be useful, but your allergy parenting decisions shouldn't be based on this type of information. When they are, you may find information that supports your doubts rather than reassures you, or you may be guided by inaccurate or unhelpful information, which unfortunately will give way to the Over-Avoidance Trap (described farther on in this chapter). Instead, whether it comes from your allergist or reputable allergic disease organizations, evidence-based information should be used whenever you're trying to answer questions (in pursuit of certainty or reassurance) or whenever you'd like to make an adjustment to how your family manages your child's allergy.

There are two main problems with seeking information from others' experiences to reassure yourself: (1) There's no right way to manage allergies, as many factors impact how families manage these diagnoses, and (2) while seeking reassurance by gathering information may initially offer a sense of control to help with uncertainty, it can result in conflicting information that adds to the confusion. A few of the many factors that influence the development of allergy management approaches include disease specifics, risk tolerance levels, family values, mindset, and past experiences. It's no surprise then that there are as many ways to parent a child with an allergy as there are colors in the big box of crayons. Therefore, your overall allergy parenting goal should be to manage your child's allergy in the best way possible for your family, given your specific circumstances and your child's specific experiences, rather than aiming to emulate what other parents do. Just because another family has the same allergic condition and a child the same age as yours doesn't mean you'll manage the condition the same way or that your child's experiences with their allergy will be the same. Using others' experiences to determine whether you're a good allergy parent can be emotionally taxing and even lead to making unnecessary changes that affect your family's quality of life. Yes, learning allergy management strategies from other parents can be useful, but when you use that information to evaluate the effectiveness of your parenting rather than to develop your own skills, the usefulness diminishes.

Finally, it's important to clarify a specific purpose or goal before engaging with social media accounts and online allergy groups. Knowing what information you're looking for and what purpose the information will serve can help keep you out of the Comparison Trap or get you out of it when feeling stuck. Don't forget to use self-imposed boundaries such as allergy-related social media breaks as needed, too. Information and online allergy groups will always be there, but you can mindfully choose when and how to engage.

Tips for getting out of the Comparison Trap:

- Know the difference between evidence-based and lived experienced–based information.
- Be accepting of the factors that make your allergy management approach good for you.
- Don't make allergy management decisions based on comparisons.
- Always discuss potential allergy management changes with your child's allergist.
- Use self-imposed boundaries such as social media breaks whenever needed.

THE CERTAINTY TRAP

Making decisions as a parent is hard and is even more complex when the outcomes directly impact your child's health and safety. As an allergy parent, you're tasked with this complex daily decision-making, which not only feels exhausting, but triggers anxiety about making the "wrong" choice that leads to an allergic reaction or asthma attack.

When stuck in the Certainty Trap, you may find yourself engaging in hours of research focused on finding clear and definitive answers that don't exist, such as what caused your child's allergy (because you believe their allergy is your fault), how to eliminate all risks (which isn't possible), and how the condition can be cured (despite no cures being available). Doing this will likely leave you feeling overwhelmed by the amount of information you feel you need to gather before making decisions, and you may even find yourself unable to trust its validity, which can induce even more anxiety. You'll also convince yourself that even a small mistake will be catastrophic or worse, fatal.

In her book *Be Mighty*, psychologist Jill Stoddard explores the anxiety triumvirate, or the three things that add fuel to the anxiety fire: (1) intolerance of uncertainty, (2) lack of perceived control, and (3) an overinflated sense of responsibility.[1] Because these three anxiety triggers are part of life with allergies, allergy parents commonly respond to them by engaging in control-seeking behaviors aimed at quieting their anxiety rather than developing allergy management skills to help navigate situations they can't control. These actions might include excessive time spent searching the Internet (to find all the answers), not letting anyone else watch your child (because only you can keep them healthy and safe), and excessive checking behaviors beyond what is necessary, such as reading labels more than a couple of times (since you worry you'll miss something). These control-seeking behaviors may initially make you feel better, but over time they can lead you to feel less in control, experience more pressure not to make any mistakes, and ultimately, make you unable to tolerate uncertainty. All of this makes parenting a child with allergies feel much harder than it needs to.

One mom reached out to me to start therapy after her child had been diagnosed with a dairy allergy and asthma because her anxiety about keeping her child safe felt overwhelming. After discussing how her anxious thoughts impacted her ability to be the allergy parent she wanted to be, it became clear that she was seeking control in order to eliminate anxiety. For example, she had made the rule that when grocery shopping, she needed to find three online sources that confirmed a product's safety before she felt certain enough to buy it. Careful label-reading and confusion about labeling laws already make grocery shopping trips long, but as you can imagine, her trips to the store took much longer, and she'd often come home without any products she felt were safe. She believed that it was possible to eliminate anxiety by feeling 100% certain about things and engaged in excessive checking behaviors in service of this. Through therapy, I helped her understand that anxiety is a normal emotional response to parenting a child with allergic conditions, that its presence doesn't always mean something bad will happen or that things are unsafe, and that the goal shouldn't be to control, fix, or avoid it. Once she leaned into this more flexible understanding about anxiety, she began taking actions to feel more prepared to navigate unexpected outcomes, such as routinely reviewing her child's emergency action plans and using empowering self-talk rather than trying to control everything. Feeling less in struggle with her anxiety, she soon noticed that her stress levels were decreasing and that decision-making didn't feel as daunting anymore.

While being doubt-free makes decision-making easier, absolute certainty is rare in life, especially life with allergies, so it's not realistic to seek 100% certainty or control. Since it's not possible to predict, identify, and control every risk, aiming to do so will only lead to further frustration and anxiety, as well as the belief that you are incapable of keeping your child safe. Throughout the COVID-19 pandemic of 2020–2023, people worldwide often found themselves in the Certainty Trap. During the shutdown phase, moms of children with food allergies felt less allergy-related anxiety despite experiencing increased generalized anxiety (associated with the inability to find safe foods and to access medical facilities safely).[2] The decrease in allergy-related anxiety was due to the increased sense of safety, as children were home where parents felt they could control experiences and outcomes. However, for many allergy parents, re-engaging in social activities post-pandemic re-triggered intense uncertainty and allergy-related anxiety, especially as they had had fewer opportunities to practice their allergy management skills outside of the home.

Ultimately, to allow your child to meet normal developmental milestones, you'll have to navigate situations that you can't control. Therefore, developing the willingness to accept that there will be uncomfortable thoughts and feelings associated with the unpredictability of allergic conditions helps you exit or stay out of the Certainty Trap. As you'll learn in later chapters, accepting this doesn't mean you have to like it, but rather, that you are willing to deal with this reality rather than trying to avoid or control it. You can begin to work toward accepting allergy-related uncertainties by taking actions that help you build confidence in your ability to manage your child's allergy. Focusing on influencing, rather than controlling outcomes is crucial when making this transition from control-seeking to skill-building. Aim to mitigate the risks you're aware of while developing strategies for safely navigating life's experiences. By regularly practicing allergy management skills as a family, preparing for a variety of situations (including identifying and addressing allergic reactions and asthma attacks), and focusing on how to navigate social scenarios and emergencies using these skills, you'll feel more capable of handling unpredictability and less engaged in control-seeking, which can give way to the Burnout Trap (discussed farther on).

Tips for getting out of the Certainty Trap

- Accept that allergy parenting includes uncertainty and unpredictability.

- Acknowledge that anxiety is a normal emotional response and doesn't need to be avoided.
- Remember that it's not possible to control every potential risk.
- Aim to influence outcomes rather than control everything.
- Practice allergy management skills and prepare for a variety of scenarios.

THE OVER-AVOIDANCE TRAP

A key allergy management tool is avoiding food-based and asthma-triggering allergens, as this helps keep allergic children healthy and safe. But what if I told you that there are times when avoidance is unhelpful? Just as you don't use a hammer for every DIY project, avoidance isn't the allergy management strategy that works best for every situation. Before I induce panic, I'm not suggesting that you put your child in unsafe situations. In fact, I'm not talking about allergen avoidance, as that's outside of my scope of practice. Rather, I'm talking about avoiding experiences and sharing evidence for why you should mindfully decide which ones to avoid rather than automatically avoid them out of fear.

While avoidance helps keep your child healthy and safe, it's also a strategy people tend to over-employ to keep from experiencing distressing thoughts and feelings, such as the ones associated with living with allergies. What's more, anxiety can drive you to overestimate risk, underestimate safety, feel certain there's an impending threat, and doubt your ability to deal with that threat, all of which can lead to excessive avoidance because everything feels unsafe. Anxious about taking your child to eat at a new restaurant? You may immediately think, *We'll just never go out to eat!* Worried that your child's asthma might be triggered if they pick up a virus at this week's story time at the library? Your initial thought might be *We'll just stay home!* Yes, avoiding those situations might feel easier—and safer—but avoiding situations just to sidestep your anxious thoughts and feelings gets in the way of developing confidence in allergy parenting. It also makes parenting a child with allergies feel harder than it should. Simply put, if you want to feel less anxious as an allergy parent, you must step outside your comfort zone and do hard things including engaging in anxiety-inducing situations (that are still safe) in service of developing and practicing allergy management skills.

Especially when you're experiencing high levels of allergy-related anxiety, your mind will likely convince you that every new situation is high risk when the actual risk levels are much lower. It also opens the door to overgeneralizations about others' experiences and outcomes and assuming that what happens to others will happen to you and your child. For instance, if your child manages asthma and another parent says that running the mile during gym triggered their son's recent asthma attack, you might find yourself believing the same will happen to your child. Or if a fellow parent of a peanut-allergic daughter shared that kissing led to an allergic reaction, you might assume that your daughter should completely avoid kissing because the same outcome will happen to her. However, it's important to remind yourself that it's normal to feel anxious hearing about others' experiences, but that your family's experiences won't necessarily be the same and that not every scenario has the same outcome.

When parents choose to avoid situations in service of keeping their child safe, that begs a key question: How exactly do you determine what's "safe enough," especially when your mind tells you that everything is potentially unsafe? You do this by using evidence-based allergen risk information and assessment strategies that will help you identify the difference between perceived (assumed) risks versus actual (confirmed) risks of allergic reactions. Ideally, all allergists would proactively educate families on how to assess and navigate allergy risks to help them determine which experiences are safe enough, but unfortunately not all do. Yet research shows that simply talking with your allergist about common fears related to the risk of allergic reactions from non-ingestion allergen exposures (e.g., touching and smelling allergens) reduces patient and parent worry about being near and touching allergens, which helps with anxiety management and can improve quality of life.[3] Alice Hoyt, a board-certified allergist, asks her patients' parents to complete the Scale of Food Allergy Anxiety (SOFAA),[4] which allows her and her team to objectively identify specific instances that are causing families stress and anxiety. Hoyt and her team then work with families to set specific goals that include the patient's personalized risks and thorough explanations of what is safe and what is not safe. While this approach is ideal, your allergist may not explore allergy-related fears as extensively. Therefore, it's important to begin these purposeful conversations with your child's allergist so you can gain insights specific to your child's allergic profile.

To help facilitate these conversations, especially if your child's allergist isn't proactively discussing allergen risk-assessment information and strategies with you, here are some key questions that I encourage you to explore with them so you can receive personalized guidance and correct potential misinformation that may be affecting your decision-making:

- How do I accurately determine what experiences or situations are too risky for my child and which ones are safe enough?
- How worried should I be about my child being near, touching, or smelling their allergen and potentially experiencing an allergic reaction or anaphylaxis as a result?
- How should I navigate precautionary allergen labeling (e.g., "may contain" and "made in a facility" warnings).
- How should I address situation-specific topics such as how to safely navigate air travel, school parties, eating out, getting vaccinations, and so on?

You'll also want to consider exploring topics such as

- strategies for safely navigating potential risks relating to food introductions, oral food challenges, and food allergy treatments, such as oral immunotherapy and sublingual immunotherapy
- any information you've found online about allergy-related risks and safety that induces anxiety and worry, excessive avoidance of situations, or that you want to fact-check.

Board-certified allergist David Stukus also shared this helpful reminder about common allergy-related overestimations of risk: "Not every allergic reaction will result in anaphylaxis, and not every episode of anaphylaxis causes fatality."[5] Similarly, not every asthma attack completely restricts airways, and respiratory failure doesn't happen every time it's difficult to breathe. In fact, despite tragic news stories about allergy-related fatalities, fatality rates aren't as high as you'd think. Recent research estimates that in the United States fewer than 100 deaths per year are due to food-induced anaphylactic reactions[6] and that these fatal reactions are less common than the risk of accidental death in the general public.[7] Asthma-related fatalities are also lower than the anxious mind suggests, with an average of 195 pediatric asthma deaths per year in the United States.[8] These statistics don't typically reassure parents because no one wants their child to be the one-in-a-million, but it's important to be aware of the data since it helps manage the allergy-related fears that can lead to over-avoidance of experiences. In addition, it's useful to remind yourself that fatality news stories initially lack specific details (since families are grieving), which can lead you to make unhelpful overgeneralizations that trigger urges to avoid similar situations that may be safe enough for your child.

You might also be avoiding discussing allergic reactions and asthma attacks with your child for fear of inducing anxiety in them. That, however, only fuels anxious "what-if" thoughts for both you and your child. Discussions, preparation, and practice combined with learning how to accurately assess allergy-related risks are key components of the Over-Avoidance Trap exit plan. Done in an age-appropriate manner, regularly reviewing your child's emergency action plan with the entire family and taking turns practicing how to calmly respond to allergic reactions and asthma attacks also helps you exit the Over-Avoidance Trap.

If your child *does* have an allergic reaction, know that it's common to initially experience increased fear and the perception that everything is unsafe. For some, these feelings persist indefinitely and unfortunately can lead to getting stuck in the Over-Avoidance trap by trying to regain control through excessive avoidance of situations. Therefore, it's useful to have a roadmap for how to navigate the often emotional and overwhelming period after reactions. To help individuals and families do this, I developed a tool called TRACE, which includes practical tips to help you mindfully re-establish balance and allergy management confidence after experiencing allergic reactions or anaphylaxis. While this information may seem like common sense, sometimes common sense escapes us when we're anxious, stressed, or traumatized, and therefore having a list of practical actions to help process and rebuild your allergy management confidence again can be very useful and empowering.

- **T**ime: It takes time to rebuild trust in your allergy management approaches again.
- **R**outine: It's helpful to get back into a normal routine as soon as possible.
- **A**llergist: Review, problem-solve, and adjust safety plans with your allergy care team.
- **C**ompassion: Be patient with and kind to yourself; find support.
- **E**ducation: Revisit allergy management information; identify and fill knowledge gaps.

(You can find a free, printable PDF version of TRACE on my resource website at www.FoodAllergyCounselor.com)

In later chapters, we'll delve deeper into specific strategies for addressing the anxious thoughts that push you to engage in over-avoidance, but for now, Table 2.1 presents basic lists

Table 2.1 Helpful Versus Unhelpful to Avoid

Helpful to Avoid	Unhelpful to Avoid
• Ingesting allergens that trigger allergic reactions, and known asthma triggers	• Anxiety, worry, or uncomfortable emotions about your child's allergy
• Foods and products without labels or an ingredient list to read through	• Skill-building opportunities so your child learns to manage their allergy
• Confirmed high-risk situations or ones where safe approaches aren't possible	• *All* new situations and experiences just because they induce anxiety and worry
• Leaving home without epinephrine autoinjectors or needle-free devices, inhalers, and other necessary emergency medications	• Practicing allergy management skills, how to use emergency medications, and reviewing emergency action plans and protocols as a family
• Making assumptions about allergy management, risks, and safety	• Discussing questions and concerns with your board-certified allergist

for when avoidance is helpful versus unhelpful in developing a more balanced, mindful approach to allergy parenting.

Tips for getting out of the Over-Avoidance Trap:

- Be aware of overgeneralizations such as "always" or "never."
- Discuss with your allergist how to do risk assessments and determine what's safe enough.
- Challenge risk overestimations and safety underestimations with evidence-based facts.
- Focus on strategies to help make situations safe enough to experience.
- Prepare for and practice skills helpful for navigating allergic reactions.

THE OVER-FUNCTIONING TRAP

With allergy parenting, one parent usually becomes the identified allergy expert—typically the parent who has the most child care responsibilities. Armed with allergic disease information and tasked with managing the day-to-day aspects, the allergy expert parent becomes almost solely responsible for their child's safety and easily gets stuck in the Over-Functioning Trap. Allergic diseases affect the whole family system, however, so management of these conditions shouldn't be only one parent's responsibility.

Parents get into the Over-Functioning Trap in a couple of ways. Sometimes it's on their own accord, in pursuit of seeking control to keep their child healthy and safe and not wanting to experience worry about trusting others to do so, including the other parent and even the allergic child. Other times, parents end up in this trap when their partner defers to them on anything allergy related, placing all the responsibility on them. No matter how they enter the Over-Functioning Trap, it's important for allergy expert parents to develop awareness of how staying stuck in this trap impacts their own functioning, their relationship with their partner, and other family members' ability to practice allergy management strategies, including the allergic child.

For the first couple years after my son was diagnosed with his food allergy, I found myself in the Over-Functioning Trap because I had become the allergy expert parent. This was because my anxious mind told me that I was the only one who knew enough about food allergies to keep my son safe. Sure, I could teach my husband and my parents all these safety strategies, but I'd still have to endure my anxious "what-if" thoughts when leaving him in their care. Yes, I was even too scared to leave my son with his own father. As you can imagine, this caused tension between my husband and me and made me feel resentful even though I was the one placing myself in this position. It also didn't help me learn to develop trust in others' ability to keep my son safe, which is a crucial component of allergy parenting as our children are in others' care as soon as they begin school.

It's probably not surprising that the addition of a child's chronic health condition, such as an allergic disease, adds another layer of complexity to parenting, which can open the door to conflict and marital discord. Allergic disease research reveals that one in four parents report that food allergies caused strain on their marriage.[9] Parents don't always see eye to eye on decisions that impact their child's health, and without effective communication and shared decision-making, ongoing tension and arguments are likely to occur. Especially when conflicts are centered on safety, such as determining what experiences are safe enough, they can trigger the protective part within the allergy expert parent. This then drives the parent further into the Over-Functioning Trap because they feel they're the only one who understands the seriousness of the allergy. It's not uncommon for this parent to also engage in one of the other parenting traps simultaneously, such as the Over-Avoidance Trap, which further supports their narrative that they're the only one who can keep their child safe. Further, this then impacts their own functioning and typically leads to the Burnout Trap, which we'll explore next.

Beyond marital strain, being stuck in the Over-Functioning Trap keeps others from learning and practicing allergy management strategies. Trusting someone means you believe in the reliability, truth, ability, and strength of another person, which can be challenging to do when it comes to caring for your child's life. Yet, the ability to trust others to keep your child safe (including the child themself) develops when you allow opportunities for the child, the other parent, and other family members to practice daily management strategies, including how to identify and respond to reactions and asthma attacks. In addition, confidence (the belief that you're good at something) develops by building competence (showing how good you are at something). As the allergy expert parent, you feel confident in your ability to keep your child safe because you've become competent in these skills over time. Your partner, child, and other family members need time and experience to do the same. Yes, you're going to fear mistakes as they practice, but remind yourself that not every mistake is catastrophic and that mistakes allow for learning and mastering skills, which helps you to become more confident in others' abilities to keep your child safe. Identify what information and skills others would need to illustrate proficiency with for you to allow them more allergy management responsibilities. Think about how you can help them develop these skills rather than avoiding opportunities to do so because of fear.

In the next chapter, we'll explore allergy parenting goals to be mindful of during various stages of allergy parenting, which will give way to caring for your child as a cohesive, balanced parental unit. This information, combined with skills you'll learn in future chapters, will help you exit the Over-Functioning Trap if you've identified yourself as the allergy expert parent taking on all the responsibility.

Tips for getting out of the Over-Functioning Trap:

- Identify if you're control-seeking or if others have placed the responsibility on you.

- Consider how over-functioning impacts your well-being, relationships, and ability to trust.
- Consider how over-functioning keeps your child from learning age-appropriate allergy management skills.
- Remember not all mistakes are catastrophic; mistakes allow for learning and skill-mastering.
- Aim to build confidence in others by allowing them to have opportunities to build competence in their allergy management skills.

THE BURNOUT TRAP

While cliché, the analogy of the candle burning at both ends fits for many allergy parents. Unlike acute illnesses that last a short time, allergic diseases persist throughout life and often include periods of acute distress after allergic reactions or asthma attacks. Meeting your child's complex health needs, keeping them safe, and navigating periods of distress all while juggling work commitments, general parenting tasks, and maintaining connections with your partner and friends is exhausting. In fact, the complexity of the parental role and parental well-being has become a growing public health issue that is being explored within allergic disease and other chronic conditions.[10]

As noted in the Over-Functioning Trap, the parent with the most child care responsibilities (often mothers) is typically identified as the allergy expert within families. Research tells us that while being highly educated about allergic conditions allows mothers to feel more empowered to care for their child's food allergies than fathers, they also report more anxiety, stress, and a greater impact on their quality of life than anyone else in the family, including their diagnosed child.[11] The allergy expert parent is often the one making health care appointments, managing and administering medications, continuously observing the child's health status, responding to emergencies, and educating others on allergies. Carrying this burden of care leads many allergy expert parents to believe they can't take a break from these responsibilities, which gives way to social isolation and parental burnout.[12] Parental burnout includes the emotional and physical exhaustion that often arises when parents endure severe stress without sufficient resources or belief in their ability to cope, which can result in feeling fed up with parenting and disengagement from the family.[13] If you're often feeling drained and unmotivated, are experiencing physical symptoms such as headaches, have trouble sleeping, and generally feel overwhelmed or resentful, you might be experiencing burnout.

Parents experiencing burnout are also often stuck in the Over-Functioning Trap, making the ongoing daily burdens too heavy to continue carrying alone. Therefore, a key strategy to help exit the Burnout Trap is to delegate allergy care and general household tasks to others in the family—even the youngest members. In her book *Autonomy-Supportive Parenting*, psychologist Emily Edlynn reminds parents that children want a sense of control over who they are and what they do (as when toddlers say, "Do it myself!") and that it's important to allow them opportunities to master skills and build competence.[14] Therefore, it's a win-win to allow children to age-appropriately become more involved in their own allergy care and general household chores since it helps them believe in their own capabilities while reducing parental burnout.

Becoming aware of your stress triggers, how your body responds to stress, and what strategies work best to manage stress also helps mitigate parental burnout. Many of the ACT-based strategies in future chapters will help you with the cognitive and emotional aspects of parental burnout, but taking care of your health in general is also important. A great place to begin is to consider the following potential burnout triggers: Are you getting enough sleep and eating foods that fuel your body? Do you spend time focusing on the other parts of yourself beyond allergy parenting? Are you able to ask for and receive help from others? Do you have a support network on this allergy parenting journey? Are you being patient with yourself, or are you setting unrealistic expectations? Each of these questions can help you begin to make adjustments that will allow you to build an exit strategy from the Burnout Trap.

Tips for getting out of the Burnout Trap:

- Notice if you're stuck in other allergy parenting traps, especially the Over-Functioning Trap.
- Delegate age-appropriate allergy care tasks and household chores whenever possible.
- Become aware of your stress triggers and symptoms and identify helpful management strategies.
- Focus on taking care of your physical and emotional health so you feel less depleted by stress.
- Be willing to ask for and receive help from others, including your children.

THE RESENTMENT TRAP

I can't tell you how many times patients and members of the allergy community have told me that the public just doesn't understand what it's like to live with allergic conditions. That's because they don't. While others can offer empathy, understanding, and compassion, people who haven't experienced living with or loving someone diagnosed with an allergic condition won't have the same perspective as those who do. This can be hard to accept.

When parents continuously experience a lack of compassion and understanding from others, they may find themselves stuck in the Resentment Trap. Resentment is a mixture of emotions including anger, frustration, bitterness, disappointment, and disgust. It's often prompted by experiencing injustices or when you are forced to accept something you don't like about someone or a situation. Resentment can also arise when you push past your own boundaries, or when you're feeling jealous or envious of others—especially those who aren't diagnosed with allergic conditions. In response to resentment, it's common to ruminate or replay things over and over in your mind, which leads to taking unhelpful actions rooted in frustration, experiencing increased stress that impacts health, and ultimately, taking an unbalanced, tunnel-vision perspective on life with allergies.

For an allergy parent, resentment due to lack of support can creep up in several places including within the family unit, school system, social circles, and the world itself. I've heard from many parents that their child's school approaches allergy care with a lack of understanding and an unwillingness to collaborate. In these scenarios, my guidance centers on finding workable solutions by asking school staff, "What *can* be done?" Resentment has a way of making people become very tunnel-visioned, so unless you're prepared to remove your child from the school, keep the endgame in mind, which is figuring out how to work together to keep your child healthy and safe while at school. Sometimes that means parents must be willing to be open-minded about how safety is achieved and possibly even adjust some requests, while staying committed to enforcing the non-negotiables (such as anaphylaxis training and having easy access to self-administered epinephrine devices and inhalers in case of emergencies). If you find that you're unable to identify which parts of a school allergy care plan should be non-negotiable versus which parts you can compromise on, have a risk-assessment discussion with your allergist to help you determine this.

I've also seen parents stuck in the Resentment Trap become overly engaged in compassion battles with people, especially on social media. Often, the goal of these compassion battles is to make others truly understand what it's like to live with allergies—an outcome that is unlikely to happen. This is especially true when debating with people who aren't open-minded or interested in showing compassion for those living with allergic conditions. Unfortunately, that drive to make people "get it" is a stressor that comes at your expense, draining your energy and time and derailing you from focusing on developing your allergy parenting skills. If you find yourself doing this, pause for a moment and evaluate where your energy is best spent—arguing with those who won't ever "get it" or channeling your energy into discussions with those who directly impact your child's safety?

How would it feel to navigate each day while wearing a very heavy backpack? Exhausting, right? Being stuck in the Resentment Trap feels like you're always carrying something that weighs you down, depletes your energy, and distracts you from your allergy parenting goals, so it's useful to find ways to set that weight down. You can start to disburden yourself of the Resentment Trap by noticing your resentment triggers, practicing gratitude for those who are understanding and supportive, setting boundaries, leaning into forgiveness, and letting go of grudges. Choosing to let go of grudges and forgiving those who are at the core of your resentment aren't about forgetting or making excuses for someone else's actions; rather, it's about shifting your energy and focus back to your needs. World-renowned researcher and author Brene Brown suggests keeping a "Damn It! Diary" to offload your resentful thoughts and to notice patterns (such as experiencing increased resentment when feeling exhausted), and then courageously set boundaries to help minimize future resentments.[15] Finally, while practicing gratitude might seem common sense, how often do you stop and think about what you're grateful for? Probably not too often. Add a few gratitude minutes to your daily schedule, and connect with the thoughts, feelings, and people who bring you joy. There are even aspects of parenting a child with allergies to be grateful for, such as learning healthier eating habits, focusing on health, and developing self-advocacy skills.

Tips for getting out of the Resentment Trap:

- Accept that not everyone will understand or show compassion for those managing allergies.

- Focus on developing workable safety solutions that might include compromise.
- Reserve your time and energy for the issues that matter and directly impact your child's safety.
- Notice what triggers your resentment and set boundaries to limit exhaustion.
- Practice gratitude, forgiveness, and letting go of grudges that no longer serve a purpose.

TAKEAWAYS

- Be aware of allergy parenting traps that lead to engaging in unhelpful behaviors and make it harder to accept and adapt to parenting a child with allergies.
- It's unhelpful to respond to the anxiety and overwhelm of allergy parenting by making comparisons, seeking complete control, avoiding discomfort and doubts, and not allowing others to help keep your child safe.
- Be sure to discuss allergy-related fears, worries, and questions with your child's allergist, as doing so often helps parents exit unhelpful allergy parenting traps.

Think About and Do

- Make a list of which traps you're stuck in, and reflect on how they're impacting you, your child, your co-parent, and your family.
- Make a separate list describing the ways in which allergy parenting would feel different for you if you weren't

stuck in these traps. What would you be able to do more or less of as a parent or as a family?

- Begin a list of allergy-related fears, worries, and questions to discuss with your child's allergist that would help you exit any parenting traps you may be stuck in. You'll likely add topics to this list as you continue reading this book.

CHAPTER 3

Setting Developmentally Focused Allergy Parenting Goals

Sam and Lisa felt overwhelmed by the reality of parenting an infant with a food allergy and found it hard to decide which allergy management information to focus on first. Shantelle struggled to say yes to playdates because it had become much harder to keep her son safe now that he was in preschool. Akira was tempted to tell her daughter that she couldn't be on the volleyball team since a handful of games were at other schools and the thought of her daughter on the bus surrounded by teammates eating snacks terrified her. Jenny often found herself losing her temper and lecturing her son about food allergy safety because of the high anxiety she had been feeling since her son began driving and spending more time with friends.

For many allergy parents, keeping their child healthy and safe while also allowing them to meet normal child developmental milestones is daunting. It may even feel impossible. How can you nurture your child's growing independence while feeling intense worry about their safety? While the ultimate parenting goal is to raise an independent and self-sufficient young adult, many wonder how it's possible to get there when simply sending your child to preschool or birthday parties feels overwhelming.

Food allergy research has explored the relationship between food allergy–related anxiety and quality of life, which is one's perception of one's general well-being and ability to participate in and enjoy life's experiences. A 2016 review summarized research illustrating that quality of life is significantly impaired for children with food allergies and their caregivers.[1] One highlighted study introduced the "Goldilocks Principle," which found that there is an optimal level of anxiety that allows for adaptive coping and effective food allergy management, while decreasing life-impacting hypervigilance, debilitating stress, and risk-taking behaviors.[2] Also referred to as a *relaxed readiness approach* to allergy management, this approach involves finding a workable level of anxiety that helps you balance vigilance and risk-taking.[3] In practical terms, a relaxed readiness approach means being aware of allergy-related risks and being ready to take action in the event of an allergic reaction, but not living in fear or, on the contrary, taking no safety precautions. Much like Goldilocks as she tried to find her "just right" porridge, chair, and bed, families managing allergies should work towards finding their "just right" relaxed readiness approach to allergy management. Consistent with previous research, this review also found that excessive parental stress and overprotective parenting practices can lead to increased anxiety and a lower quality of life for an allergic child. Yet while the benefits of approaching allergies with relaxed readiness are apparent, doing so is often hard to put into practice, especially because every family's "just right" balance between fear and living fully looks different.

As I thought through the stages of allergy parenthood and the goal of taking a relaxed readiness approach to allergy management, I felt that additional guidance was needed to help parents figure out how to adopt this approach. This led me to discover the research of Ellen Galinsky, who conducted interviews with hundreds of parents and found that parents of all cultural and socioeconomic backgrounds went through similar parenthood stages that coincided with their children's development. Her theory is that parents develop as their children grow and that as parents enter each new stage of their child's development, their role as parents changes, too.[4] I realized that allergy parents needed guidance on how their roles change and what they themselves should be focused on accomplishing during each stage of their child's development, as this could help them develop effective approaches for being vigilant while also being mindful of development. Because keeping your child healthy and safe is a cornerstone in allergy parenting, it's easy to focus only on allergy management and forget to nurture the child and parental developmental processes, too. Yet, it's important to learn how to pay attention to all developmental processes if you want to work toward a balanced, relaxed readiness approach to life with allergies.

The insights shared in this chapter can help you stay mindful of three key developmental processes (child, parental, and allergy management) within each age and stage—infancy, toddlerhood and preschool, middle childhood, and adolescence and young adulthood. For each stage, we'll look at the overall parenting goals, allergy parenting tasks on which to focus, emotional responses that can derail the developmental processes, and important conversations to have. Remember that while anxiety often pushes us to avoid things that make us worry, avoiding key allergy parenting tasks to calm your own anxiety can make future ages and stages harder for you and your child. Children learn best through scaffolding, or learning over time with age-appropriate assistance in building on previously mastered tasks with new skills. Therefore, think of each stage of your child's development as the foundation for the next stage, in which they will expand on their current skills. Also, keep in mind that the ultimate allergy parenting goal is to help your child learn how to effectively manage their own allergy and to engage in a balanced, relaxed readiness approach to life with allergies.

Not everything in this chapter will feel like a perfect fit for everyone, and that's okay. This guidance should be applied with the specifics of your family in mind, including your child's maturity level and allergic disease specifics. As always, discuss any and all of your concerns with your child's board-certified allergist and allergy care team.

INFANCY

Parents' Role and Overall Goal

New to the world, infants begin developing trust in the care that their parents provide as soon as they're born. For parents, the overall goal during this stage is to adapt to life as a parent and to develop an attachment with the baby. This includes accepting the realities of life as a parent, which may not align with what you had expected, as well as learning more about yourself as you step into this new role. Because parents are fully responsible for their child's health and safety at this age, even beyond allergic conditions, parents act as *protectors*. When allergic conditions are diagnosed during this stage, it only intensifies what might already be an overwhelming transition.

Allergy Parenting Goals and Tasks to Focus On

As shared in previous chapters, it's not uncommon to feel overwhelmed, frustrated, and worried after your child receives their diagnosis, which for many, happens during infancy and toddlerhood. The main allergy parenting goals in this stage are to work toward accepting your child's allergy diagnosis and adapting to daily life with allergies. Accepting your child's diagnosis doesn't mean you have to like it—who does? Rather, to accept the diagnosis means having the willingness to make room for all the thoughts and feelings that arise, even the painful and uncomfortable ones, and to continue to engage in meaningful experiences. Without learning how to accept your child's allergies, which we'll explore more in future chapters, you may find yourself resisting, running from, or fighting with uncomfortable thoughts and feelings, which typically makes the overwhelm feel worse. It's common to want to resist accepting reality when reality brings with it pain. Yet, as you'll continue to learn throughout this book, acceptance is a key component of reducing the overwhelm of allergy parenting, developing a balanced approach that isn't led by fear, and teaching your child the necessary skills to become a self-sufficient young adult.

Adapting to life with allergies begins by learning what the diagnosis means and how it impacts everyday life, as well as developing your own strategies for keeping your child healthy and safe. Overwhelmed with fear, many parents feel like they need to become sponges after receiving their child's diagnosis—ready to absorb as much information as quickly and humanly possible to keep their child safe. Yet, if you try to learn everything all at once, you'll become like a waterlogged sponge—too full and overwhelmed to do your job effectively. When Sam and Lisa received their son's egg allergy diagnosis, they both felt frozen with fear and grief at the same time that they felt the desire to learn as much as they could about keeping their son safe. Neither could believe that their son had been diagnosed with a food allergy. Sam started drafting follow-up questions for their son's allergist, while Lisa began searching every food allergy–related website she could find. Every moment Lisa wasn't researching food allergy management strategies, her mind told her that she wasn't being a good enough allergy parent. Yet, the more time she spent online, the more anxious and overwhelmed she became, and the harder it was to settle into managing her son's egg allergy. She desperately wanted to adjust to life with a food allergy as quickly as possible but was burning herself out in the process.

Learning how to live with allergic conditions takes time and experience, so overwhelming yourself with too much information too quickly only hinders the adjustment process. Therefore, consider using the *PACED approach* to navigate opinions and information in such a way that you can feel empowered rather than overwhelmed:

Prioritize present-focused topics.
Assess the source of information.
Confirm information with your allergist.
Evaluate insights offered by others carefully.
Decide daily management strategies first.

The PACED approach encourages you to stay focused on gathering information for priority topics, such as daily management strategies and anything that relates to navigating your child's current stage of development. It also emphasizes the importance of understanding and evaluating the source of information and opinions you're receiving, especially when it comes to lived experience and insights from others, which can easily lead to your second-guessing how you're managing your child's allergy. This approach also emphasizes how important it is to confirm information with your child's allergist before making decisions and major shifts in allergy management. The best place to turn to for reliable information is your child's board-certified allergist, as they are specialists in allergy and immunology and are also familiar with your child's specific allergies. If you don't trust your allergist's guidance, then it's a good idea to seek out a second opinion, because a trusting relationship with your child's allergist is crucial to the process of accepting and adapting to life with allergies. While you may feel too overwhelmed to think of and ask questions at the diagnosis appointment—which is understandable—write down any questions and concerns that arise while processing the information so that you can follow up with your child's allergist to get evidence-based information that will help you adjust to life with allergies. One allergist friend recently told me, "I'd rather have parents reach out to me with questions than spend hours online trying to find answers that may not even be accurate and may make allergy management more difficult." So, truly, don't hesitate to reach out to your child's allergist with questions, even if you think they're silly ones.

For parents of children managing food allergy, I also recommend using the American Academy of Allergy, Asthma & Immunology's "Food Allergy Stages Handouts" and allergist Scott Sicherer's *The Complete Guide to Food Allergies in Adults and Children* for additional evidence-based insights and allergy management strategies.[5] You'll also want to find support networks, as connecting with other families who manage the same condition will help you accept and adapt to the diagnosis. At the same time, be mindful of whether others' opinions and having a constant focus on allergies are exacerbating the overwhelm you're experiencing rather than helping it.

Be Mindful Of

During each stage, it's important to pay attention to any unhelpful narratives, mindsets, and allergy parenting traps mentioned in previous chapters, as they will contribute to the overwhelm, particularly as you're entering life with allergies. Parents of infants managing allergic conditions can easily get trapped in the Certainty, Over-Avoidance, and Over-Functioning Traps in service of seeking control and eliminating all risk rather than prioritizing information-gathering, conversations with their allergist, and practicing allergy management skills. This is because we tend to engage in actions that calm our anxiety in the short term without thinking about the long-term impact those actions may have.

With food allergies, an example of an unhelpful, but common action, which is meant to quiet parental anxiety in the short term, but which can lead to negative long-term impacts, is avoiding food introductions. Yet research shows that early introduction of allergens can help with the prevention of food allergies,[6] as well as help to ensure that children are receiving adequate, balanced nutrition. Especially when there's an older sibling already managing a food allergy, parental anxiety about introducing allergens to subsequent siblings allows versions of this common "what-if" question to get in the way: *What if my older child reacts because we have his allergen in the house to introduce to my younger child?* This fear can lead to other food introduction struggles such as waiting for the perfect day to introduce foods (there isn't one), believing you must feel calm rather than anxious to successfully introduce foods (it's normal for anxiety to be present when doing something new), and experiencing complete overwhelm about how to get started with food introductions. If you're nodding your head in agreement as you read these statements, you're not alone. Many parents who are at this stage are anxious about food introductions, but the key is to develop a workable plan that helps you to follow through and continue to incorporate tolerated allergens in your child's diet. Think about what might be helpful for these introductions, such as having a support person with you, doing them when your older child is out of the house, and making an introduction schedule that works best for you. Be sure to discuss any and all concerns and worries with your child's allergist to receive practical information and guidance that will likely help you address your allergen introduction fears.

Another example of an action that is meant to calm anxiety but that often does the reverse is thinking too far in the future to prepare for everything possible in your child's life. This leads to anticipatory anxiety, which keeps you from functioning optimally in your current stage of parenting. It also not only exacerbates overwhelm but can impact your ability to meet the basic developmental needs of this stage, which include establishing the parent-child relationship and becoming the parent you want to be. My own story from the introduction chapter illustrated that I wasn't initially willing to accept my son's peanut allergy and instead ruminated over every future-focused "what-if." My mind wanted to envision every possible life experience he'd have in order to prepare for and protect myself from more pain in the future.

It was only when I became willing to sit with sadness, grief, and anger—acknowledging that it was normal for those feelings to be present and that I didn't have to do anything with them other than feel them—that I was able to stop engaging with all of the future-focused worries, accept his diagnosis (which I couldn't change anyhow), and take purposeful action aimed at adjusting to life with my son's peanut allergy.

Talk About

Conversations between you and your co-parent should explore general parenting approaches, especially if you're new to parenthood, such as defining what kind of allergy parents you want to be and creating a shared vision for how you want to manage your child's allergy. Consider doing the following with your partner and/or co-parent:

- Develop a list of follow-up questions for your child's allergist, which should include questions about daily allergy management and how to manage fears about your child's health and safety so that these fears don't keep your family from important experiences.
- Establish your family's allergy management routines. If you are unable to reach a shared decision about how to manage your child's allergies, reach out to your child's allergist to gather more information.
- Identify what might be impacting your ability to accept the diagnosis and/or fueling your anxiety. Be honest about what you need from one another physically and emotionally as you adjust to life with allergies.
- Identify each other's strengths and discuss how each of you can use these strengths to help the family adjust to life with allergies.

TODDLERHOOD AND PRESCHOOL

Parents' Role and Overall Goal

The child's world expands as they're on the go and exposed to more experiences as a toddler and preschooler. Developmental goals in this stage are focused on developing skills that lead to building a sense of personal control and age-appropriate autonomy. Children also begin learning how to navigate complex feelings such as shame and doubt, which can impact confidence-building, the willingness to try new things, and how they feel about themselves. Acting as *leaders*, parents focus on teaching rules and guiding the child's behavior, while at the same time allowing the child to engage in age-appropriate separation and independence. As a result, there are lots of instances of "No!" and "I do it!" as parents often experience power struggles while the child tests boundaries to determine the rules.

Allergy Parenting Goals and Tasks to Focus On

During the toddlerhood and preschool years, you're still responsible for your child's overall safety and health, but you will begin teaching your child age-appropriate allergy management strategies. Just as you teach your child to look both ways and to hold an adult's hand before crossing the road, you can (and should) begin teaching your young child allergy basics. Having done your own work to accept and adapt to life with allergies will make it easier to help your child accept their diagnosis as they observe how you manage it in various experiences outside of your home. Their growing curiosity and desire to be active may make you feel anxious about keeping them safe in new experiences, but consider the flip side—namely, their age-appropriate need for autonomy. With toddlers and preschoolers being willing and excited to learn and try new things, you have an abundance of opportunities to teach your child foundational allergy management skills to build upon in future stages.

Teaching your child how to age-appropriately understand their allergy and begin navigating life with it requires the willingness to engage in new experiences inside and outside of the home, such as playdates and park excursions, where you both can practice new skills that help build competence and confidence. Shantelle's son loved preschool and had made lots of new friends whose parents regularly scheduled playdates at each other's houses. Because she had just settled into the new preschool routine, she felt intense anxiety when her son began getting invited to playdates. She found herself torn between wanting to say no because she feared for his safety in someone else's home and wanting to say yes because she saw how excited her son was when playing with his new friends. Unsure what to do, we discussed the pros and cons of each option and explored what she would choose to do if her anxiety wasn't getting in the way. With gentle encouragement, Shantelle also scheduled a consultation call with her son's allergist to discuss her fears about the risks of attending playdates in others' homes. The allergist validated Shantelle's feelings, explored risk-assessment strategies, discussed communicating safety routines with other parents, and encouraged her to use these playdates as food allergy teachable moments with her son. While still anxious, Shantelle tapped into this new roadmap as she gave playdates a try and found that doing so was empowering for both her and her son.

Rather than responding to the overwhelm by leaning into worry, focus on the skills you want your child to master, including knowing that they have an allergy, being aware of their food allergen or asthma triggers, and learning basic allergy safety rules, such as washing hands and asking an adult if it's safe before eating anything. These basics also include teaching them the name of their food allergens (through photos, pictures, toys, and stories), helping them learn basic terms such as "safe" and "not safe," learning how to tell others about their allergy and to speak up if their body doesn't feel right, and identifying their emergency medications. Be creative in how you teach these skills. Using play-based strategies such as songs, role-playing, storytelling, and make-believe play with stuffed animals will make it more fun for both you and your child. Asking more experienced allergy parents how they taught their young child about their allergy can expand your list of strategies as well.

During this stage, your child might start expressing big feelings such as sadness and disappointment if they have to miss out on an experience such as a birthday party, a delicious dessert, or an outing. This is especially true for children with allergic conditions as they tend to experience disappointment from a young age. As parents, we want to shield our children from pain or struggle. While doing so might feel like a relief, it's unrealistic to think that we can keep them from these feelings since we don't have control over every experience they'll have. What's more, kids need to learn how to deal with disappointment. An effective way to teach them to do so is by noticing, naming, and talking about the emotions they feel, rather than doing what might feel easiest—avoiding any experience that makes them feel sad.

Be Mindful Of

Experiences outside of the home are important for toddlers and preschoolers, as they help them learn about the world around them and begin to understand how to navigate a variety of experiences with their allergy. Especially if you're stuck in the Over-Functioning and Over-Avoidance Traps, you may be unwilling to engage in experiences that will help you develop trust in others' ability to care for your child, such as leaving your child in the care of family members or babysitters. This can lay the foundation for how the child views their ability to stay safe outside of their home or with anyone besides you (*I'm not safe anywhere but home or with my parents*) and can make it harder for both you and your child to transition to the next stage when your child is out of the home during full-day school.

Be mindful of how your own anxiety is affecting your actions in other areas as well. It may push you to avoid allowing and encouraging your child to try new foods, which can further impact eating patterns and mealtime behaviors. Especially for children managing food allergies and food-based allergic conditions, it's important to help them develop a healthy relationship with food and the ability to focus on what they *can* eat, not just what they can't eat. A dad who was a guest on my "Exploring Food Allergy Families" podcast shared that after his son was initially diagnosed with multiple food allergies, he found himself thinking about all the foods and meals his son couldn't have. Soon after the diagnosis, he attended a local food allergy support group meeting whose guest speaker encouraged parents to make two lists: a list of foods that their child couldn't eat AND a list of foods their child could eat. He shared that creating the "can eat" list felt empowering and helped him shift his perspective from focusing solely on the negatives to focusing on the possibilities, too.

Talk About

Conversations between you and your co-parent should focus on how you'll adjust your allergy management approaches to safely nurture your child's growing curiosity and preparing for others to care for your child, whether at home or at preschool. With your child, it's useful to set the stage for talking about how they feel about their allergy and helping them learn words for expressing their emotions. Consider doing the following with your partner and/or co-parent:

- Decide strategies for teaching your child allergy basics, as well as what language, tone, and narratives you'll use when talking about the allergy (and allergic reactions or asthma attacks) in their presence.
- Decide what allergy management routines you'll educate others about (e.g., babysitter, family members, teachers, other parents), especially if they'll be caring for your child.
- Discuss what conversations to have with your allergist that will help you make decisions about specific transitional concerns as your child enters preschool (e.g., assessing allergy-related risk levels of school activities, educating teachers, providing safe snacks, identifying allergens in the school environment).
- Identify important experiences you want your family to engage in even while managing allergies and identify emotional and fear-based roadblocks getting in the way of doing so.
- Consider reaching out to a mental health professional if you and/or your co-parent notice anxiety that impacts daily functioning and your ability to nurture your child's development.

MIDDLE CHILDHOOD

Parents' Role and Overall Goal

As children move through elementary school and into their preteen years, their sense of self continues to develop. Facing new challenges and social experiences, they'll have opportunities to practice new emotional and social skills. During this stage, children are learning how to receive feedback from teachers and coaches, work through conflicts with friends, and persevere even when they're not feeling confident. When children aren't given opportunities to develop and practice these age-appropriate skills, they may come to believe that they're less capable than their peers.

Consequently, during this stage, parents act as *guides*, helping their child interpret and make sense of social experiences and the world around them. This requires having the willingness to answer questions, provide information, teach skills, and help your child formulate values (what they want to stand for), which will guide them as they develop their confidence and self-worth.[2] Keeping in mind that the next stage of development is adolescence—a time when children want growing independence, responsibility, and more space away from you—you should remind yourself that skills learned during this stage helps both you and your child with that big developmental transition.

Allergy Parenting Goals and Tasks to Focus On

A main allergy parenting goal during this stage is to help your child nurture their social health (friendships and community) while practicing necessary skills for managing their allergy and keeping themselves safe, especially while outside of the home. At this age, children should become more involved in allergy management beyond the basics. In the early elementary years and with your supervision, they can follow safety routines, help with label-reading, say no to unsafe foods, tell a trusted adult when they're experiencing uncomfortable physical sensations, and possibly even carry their own emergency medications. In the later elementary and middle school years, these skills should expand to include involvement in food preparation, practicing how to navigate social outings safely, teaching their friends about their allergies, having a deeper understanding of the symptoms of allergic reactions and asthma attacks, and developing routines to remember their emergency medications. Decisions on when and how to include your child in their allergy management should be guided by the following factors: (1) your child's level of maturity, (2) their willingness to gain responsibility, and (3) their ability to put the allergy management skills they've been taught into action. Some children may be ready to carry their own self-administered epinephrine devices and inhalers by first grade (even if they're not ready to use them on their own), while others may not be ready until the end of elementary school. Children who are outgoing may find it easier to self-advocate at birthday parties from a young age, while those who are shy may struggle to do so until they're older. You know your child best.

As scary as it might feel to allow your child to become more hands-on (and for you to pull back in some areas), it's important for you to do so for your child's development. While the thought of your child possibly making mistakes feels overwhelming—especially when thinking of worst-case scenarios—remember that avoiding experiences just to control your anxiety keeps your child from practicing necessary allergy management skills and may inadvertently teach them that they're incapable of learning how to keep themselves safe. Instead, lead with empowering messages such as "This may feel hard at first, so let's keep practicing!" and model for them (and yourself) that allergies are manageable when you prepare, take precautions, have emergency medications, and know your emergency action plan.

As your child continues to navigate new social experiences, it's helpful to proactively explore a variety of social scenarios that your child might experience and teach more advanced self-advocacy and assertive communication skills, especially if they're shy. Whether it's through conversations or engaging in role-playing, explore both easy and challenging social situations. Easier social situations might include asking safety questions such as ingredient lists, politely turning down food offers, responding to curious peers asking questions about their allergy such as "Why can't you eat the same snack as me?" or "Why do you cough after you run?," and teaching their friends about their allergy. In fact, children and teens often report that having friends who are understanding and supportive of their allergy helps them feel more comfortable engaging in health-promoting behaviors.[7] More challenging social situations to explore might include what to do if your child feels excluded, teased, or bullied because of their allergy. One in three children managing food allergy and one in ten children managing asthma reported that they've experienced allergy-related bullying.[8] Therefore, it's important to proactively talk about how to respond to and seek help from an adult in these instances. In addition, encourage your child not to feel ashamed or embarrassed of their allergy, and help them understand that it's just one part—among many—that makes them who they are.

Be Mindful Of

Any time there's a transition in life, such as when your child enters a new developmental stage, it's understandable to notice an uptick in anxiety and worry. As your child spends more time outside of the home (and away from your supervision), pay attention to what's increasing your own anxiety, any unhelpful thoughts and narratives that are leading you into allergy parenting traps, and the actions you're taking as a result. For instance, it's easy to end up in the Over-Avoidance Trap in these middle childhood years by requesting accommodations at school beyond what's medically necessary or age-appropriate for your child simply to calm your fears. Maybe your child now wants to sit with their friends at lunch rather than sitting at the allergy-friendly table, which they've done since kindergarten. Even if your child's allergist offers guidance on safe strategies for doing so, your fear may push you to say no to this transition. However, consider this: While keeping your child at the allergy-friendly table may indefinitely decrease your own anxiety, it might limit your child's ability to develop and practice their own allergy management skills. It may also impact their friendships and social health, leading your child to feel more socially excluded than their allergy already makes them feel.

When I began working with Akira, she was on the verge of telling her sixth-grade daughter that she couldn't join the volleyball team since a handful of the games were at other schools. The thought of her daughter on a bus filled with snacks that included her allergens felt incredibly scary. Yet,

Akira also recognized that her daughter was very mature for her age and was already managing her food allergies well without much input from her. After exploring how saying no would calm her own fears but at her daughter's expense—it would impact her daughter's social health and ability to continue expanding her allergy management skills—Akira decided to allow her daughter to join the volleyball team and focused her energy on ensuring that her daughter was prepared ahead of each game and ready to use her self-administered epinephrine device if needed.

Your anxiety may also keep you from talking with your child about allergic reactions and asthma attacks for fear of making them anxious. Even though avoiding these conversations may temporarily decrease your anxiety, doing so tells your child that allergic reactions and asthma attacks are scary—too scary to even talk about. How does that help your child learn to identify and prepare to respond to reactions? It doesn't. In fact, avoiding these conversations can breed anxiety and prevent you and your child from developing trust in your emergency medications and action plans, neither of which is helpful. Instead, teach your child the emergency action basics: how to calmly notice concerning symptoms and physical sensations within their body (to help them learn how to identify an allergic reaction or asthma attack) and how to communicate these concerns to trusted adults who can help them respond with emergency medications. Practice these routines regularly to help your child understand that their medication and action plans are important tools for keeping them healthy and safe. In addition, because children pick up on their parents' tone of voice and body language, be mindful of the way in which you talk about allergic reactions and asthma attacks in front of them. Especially for children who tend to feel anxious, it's unhelpful for them to listen to intense reaction stories or hear you using scary language such as "life-threatening" to refer to their allergy. Yes, they need to understand the serious nature of their allergy, but this can be conveyed in an age-appropriate manner without using scary language. Saying "Peanuts can make your body very sick" is much less anxiety-inducing to hear than "Peanuts can kill you." These conversations are additional situations where balance is needed—a balance between educating your child and doing so age-appropriately and in a way that doesn't induce high anxiety that impairs their daily functioning.

Talk About

Conversations between you and your co-parent should focus on preparing your child to navigate a variety of new situations, helping them interpret social experiences, and developing a sense of resiliency. With your child, it's useful to continue making space for them to talk about how they feel about their allergy and to problem-solve situations together. Consider doing the following with your child:

- Encourage your child to share any questions or concerns they have about their allergy.
- Encourage your child to identify how well they're managing their allergy.
- Help your child develop empowering thoughts as they learn how to manage their allergy.
- Use a team approach for preparing ahead of new situations, especially if your child is worried.

- If your child experiences an allergic reaction or asthma attack, help them return to normal routines and process what went well and what you'll do differently going forward.
- Identify and practice emotional coping skills with the child—and/or as a family—to help manage anticipatory anxiety as you and your child continue engaging in new experiences. This might include taking deep, calming breaths and writing/drawing about feelings.
- Consider reaching out to a mental health professional if you notice your child's anxieties or worries are impacting their functioning and willingness to engage in new experiences.

ADOLESCENCE AND YOUNG ADULTHOOD

Parents' Role and Overall Goal

The adolescent years are the final steppingstone from childhood to young adulthood. This phase can feel daunting for many parents—and for teenagers themselves—because it includes significant physical, social, and emotional development. The main developmental tasks for teenagers and young adults are to gain a better understanding of who they are and to work toward acquiring the skills necessary to live and function on their own in the future. Essentially, your teenager or young adult is developing their own identity—one that may differ from how you see them. They're examining their own beliefs, values, and thoughts while trying to understand how they fit in (or don't fit in) with peers, family, and the world around them.

Throughout this stage and into young adulthood, the teenage brain goes through a maturation process that involves neurochemical changes that are meant to encourage maturity, but that can lead to engaging in risky behaviors since teens tend to weigh positive experiences more heavily than negative ones.[9] This is because while the pre-frontal cortex, or the part of the brain involved in problem-solving, impulse-control, and judgement, continues developing into young adulthood, this maturation process can be impacted by physical, mental, behavioral, and environmental factors. As a result, teen logic doesn't always make sense—or feel reassuring—to parents and may lead to increased conflict in the parent-child relationship.

To allow these normal developmental processes to happen, parents act as *coaches* during the adolescent years with the goal of becoming even more hands-off during young adulthood. Your role as the coach is to encourage your teen to engage in critical thinking and problem-solving, to facilitate two-way conversations (where you listen as much, if not more, than you talk), to continue teaching them self-efficacy skills, and to be there as a support when they make mistakes along the way, which they will. These tasks may feel easy to achieve one day and incredibly hard the next day, especially when allergies are added to the equation.

Allergy Parenting Goals and Tasks to Focus On

The overall allergy parenting goal with teenagers is to help them develop their ability to make safe and appropriate decisions, while avoiding overly cautious and avoidant behaviors that negatively impact their social, emotional, and physical functioning. It's helpful to remember that children learn best when learning includes age-appropriate assistance and opportunities to practice over time as they work to acquire new skills. This means that all the allergy management skills you've helped your child learn in the previous developmental phases provides them with a solid foundation to build upon and the ability to manage their allergy more effectively during the teen and young adulthood years.

It's probably no surprise that the adolescent years tend to be one of the most anxiety-inducing developmental periods for allergy parents, as teenagers and parents often don't see eye to eye on allergy management during this stage. It literally feels like you're playing safety tug of war at times. While allergic teenagers and young adults want to experience normal development by gaining more independence, spending more time outside of the home, and pursuing activities that feel rewarding, allergy parents often worry that they'll make unsafe choices and/or will hesitate to use emergency medications, especially if they're not yet exhibiting responsible behaviors or tend to give in to peer pressure to avoid embarrassment. That's why it's even more crucial in this stage to act as the *coach*, allowing your teenager opportunities to practice skills, make mistakes, and manage challenges with your guidance. Doing so also allows you and your teenager to build trust: You're letting them know that you're willing to trust them at the same time they're learning to trust their own allergy management capabilities.

In the case of food allergy, parents have good reason to be concerned about their allergic teenager's safety. Research shows that fatal food-induced anaphylaxis is most likely to occur during adolescence and young adulthood in part due to the developmental and transitional changes occurring.[10] I'm sure reading that kicked your anxiety level up a notch—that's completely understandable. While the overall food allergy fatality rates are low even within this age group, no parent wants their child to be a statistic. Trust me when I say you're not alone. Remember, I'm not only a licensed therapist, but also the parent of a teenager managing a peanut allergy, so I often feel anxious about navigating this developmental stage, too. These fears and worries about safety are what make it very difficult to find balance between all the developmental processes happening simultaneously (your teen's, your own, and allergy management). Yet, it's also what makes finding balance so critically important, because, simply stated, our teenagers must learn how to manage their allergies on their own, and that happens through practice. Therefore, rather than ruminating over the many "what-ifs" of parenting an allergic teenager and young adult, let's explore parenting tasks that involve a balanced approach, allowing our teenagers to build necessary self-efficacy skills while also making sure they're safe.

Allergy parenting tasks during adolescence and young adulthood tend to fall under three categories: *allergy education, allergy management*, and *health management and navigation*. Specific parenting tasks in each of these categories will help teenagers learn how to effectively understand and navigate important allergy management responsibilities on their own.

For evidence-based information guiding these recommendations, check out the following resources: (1) the previously mentioned AAAAI's "Food Allergy Stages Handouts," (2) *Allergies and Adolescents: Transitioning Towards Independent Living*, edited by David Stukus,[11], and (3) a position paper entitled "A Practical Toolbox for the Effective Transition of Adolescents and Young Adults with Asthma and Allergies" produced by the European Academy of Allergy and Clinical Immunology.[12]

Achieving these tasks doesn't happen overnight. It takes time and practice. Remember, too, that you're not tasked with helping your teenager learn and develop these necessary self-management skills on your own. That should be a joint effort between you, your teenager, and your allergist.

Allergy Education and Allergy Management

It's not uncommon for teenagers and young adults to coast when it comes to living with allergies, especially if they have not had an allergic reaction or asthma attack in years. By this age, they know the allergy basics, what they must do to stay healthy and safe, and have been practicing allergy management skills for a while (one hopes). Even so, there are often allergy knowledge and skills gaps during this stage, along with allergy care topics that need to be revisited and/or expanded on. As young children, they receive lots of allergy management education from you as they begin learning how to live with their allergy, but this education often slows (or even stops) as they start getting older. That, however, can be concerning. In fact, it's important for parents to see adolescence as a stage that requires *more* education and skill-building, not less.

Key *allergy education* topics to revisit and expand upon include

- reviewing food avoidance and making safe food choice options
- reviewing asthma triggers and choices to reduce the likelihood of an asthma attack

- reviewing the symptoms of allergic reactions and asthma attacks
- reviewing food allergy and asthma emergency action plans, including discussing what actions to take for mild versus severe reactions, as well as what to do if symptoms worsen or don't get better after using a self-administered epinephrine device or an inhaler
- reviewing the importance of utilizing rescue and reliever medications in a timely manner as instructed by their allergist and regularly practice using each of these.

Key *allergy management* topics to revisit and expand on include

- reviewing and practicing assertive communication skills (especially with shy teenagers) and how to self-advocate with peers, teachers, coaches, and health care professionals
- exploring how and when they should disclose information about their allergy and educate their peers and other trusted adults so that others can help them identify allergy-related risks, stay safe, and respond to reactions if necessary
- discussing the benefits of engaging in risk-reduction behaviors whenever possible, focusing on how to do so while still having fun, as well as the costs of not paying attention to allergy-related risks and the impacts that can have on social experiences
- identifying and discussing how to deal with common potential allergy management risks in social situations,

including eating out, navigating peer pressure (including drugs and alcohol, which can further impair judgement), dating, kissing, and traveling

- identifying and discussing the benefits and costs of common teenage risk-taking behaviors, including not carrying self-administered epinephrine devices or inhalers, not preparing prior to social outings (especially ones involving food), not assessing and avoiding allergy-related risks in the moment, and not being willing to use self-administered epinephrine devices and inhalers if having an allergic reaction or asthma attack to avoid embarrassment in front of peers
- discussing decision-making about future college and career choices that allow them to manage their allergy safely.

Health Management and Navigation

Teenagers who manage allergies will be required to learn health management and navigation skills earlier than those who don't have chronic conditions. They'll need to know who their doctors are, how to fill out health care forms, how to refill medications, and how to find emergency services. Teenagers may push back on their parents about needing to learn these skills, especially if their peers aren't being taught them, but it's important to emphasize that these are skills all young adults eventually need to learn and to stay the course with your teenager.

Key *health management and navigation* topics to revisit and expand upon include

- providing them with written information about their medical history, past allergic reactions and asthma attacks, medications, and overall health profile

- offering them guidance on how to talk with their allergist and letting them practice taking charge during their health care appointments
- teaching them how to understand and complete health care forms, paying special attention to consent forms
- reviewing medications and expiration dates and teaching them how to renew prescriptions
- encouraging them to pay attention to their mental health and teaching them how to locate a mental health professional if they need emotional support.

Be Mindful Of

As with the other developmental stages, it's important to be mindful of your own anxiety levels. Remember, how you choose to manage your own anxiety can directly impact your teenager's ability to develop necessary self-management skills, which only increases your anxiety about their ability to stay safe and their own beliefs about being capable of keeping themselves safe.

Especially in adolescence, it's beneficial to take a *shared decision-making approach* when making major decisions or changes relating to your teenager's allergy. In health care, shared decision-making is an evidence-based approach in which patients and doctors work together to decide a care plan that incorporates patients' preferences, goals, and values.[13] It's always beneficial to work collaboratively with your allergist, but especially as you navigate adolescent allergy management transitions. Doing so not only leads to developing the best care plan for your teenager and your family, but also allows your teenager to experience patient-centered care so that they will continue to seek out doctors who engage in shared decision-making when they are adults.

In addition, be mindful of how you'll respond when your teenager makes allergy management mistakes, because they likely will. Making mistakes is part of the learning process, especially when acquiring new skills. Yes, they may even make big mistakes that result in allergic reactions or asthma attacks, and those mistakes are hard pills to swallow as an allergy parent. (Adolescence is a good time to remind yourself of these important statements shared in Chapter 2: *Not every allergic reaction will result in anaphylaxis, and not every episode of anaphylaxis causes fatality. Similarly, not every asthma attack completely restricts airways, and respiratory failure doesn't happen every time it's difficult to breathe.*) Is it okay to let your teenager know if you're disappointed in their decisions? Absolutely. Part of the learning process, especially at this age, is what happens after making a mistake—reviewing the experience, receiving feedback, and then coming up with new approaches or solutions. Given that your goal is to help your teenager develop their critical thinking skills, your tone and approach to conversations about mistakes matters. Approaching them with an angry, judgmental tone (likely fueled by anxiety about their choices) will only shut down conversations. That's exactly what happened when Jenny began lecturing her son about the importance of food allergy management because she was so anxious about the possibility of him making poor choices and having an allergic reaction. Her son felt like she assumed he would make poor choices just because he was a teenager, even when he hadn't given her any reason to believe he would. As a result, he started tuning her out and stopped sharing information with her, which only increased her anxiety. Once she became aware of how her approach was impacting her son, she quickly pivoted and began addressing her anxiety so that she could approach these discussions with her son calmly. As Jenny learned, be prepared to process your feelings before talking with your teenager so that you can approach them calmly, too.

Talk About

Conversations with your teenager or young adult should focus on helping them deepen their allergy management skills, communication strategies, and ability to navigate the world with their allergy. It's easy to forget to listen when you want to make sure that your teenager is taking their allergy seriously, but remember to listen as much—if not more—than you talk when discussing allergy management topics with them. Consider doing the following with your teenager:

- Focus on allowing your teenager opportunities to develop their critical thinking skills by asking questions such as "What would you do in this situation?" rather than immediately telling them what to do.
- Explore upcoming transitions, including transitions to high school, college, and the workforce, openly sharing your thoughts and concerns with each other.
- Ask them to share their thoughts and feelings about trying to balance being a teenager and keeping themselves safe and explore what is working well and not working well for them.
- Talk about the importance of having a growth mindset and believing that you can learn how to manage your allergy even if it feels overwhelming at first.

- Help them learn and use coping strategies if they're experiencing allergy-related anxiety and discuss the benefits of talking with a mental health professional if they want additional support.

TAKEAWAYS

- One key goal in allergy parenting is to work toward developing a relaxed readiness approach, which will allow you and your family to manage allergy-related anxiety so you can meaningfully engage in life's experiences while also being ready to respond to allergic reactions if necessary.
- Another key goal in allergy parenting is to find a workable balance between the three developmental processes happening at the same time: your child's development, your parental development, and the development of allergy management skills.
- Focusing on your child's current stage of development helps make allergy parenting overwhelm feel more manageable. Yet it's also important to stay mindful of the ultimate allergy parenting goal that you're working toward: raising a self-sufficient young adult who can effectively manage and navigate the world with their allergy.

Think About and Do

- Notice if you often find yourself anxiously focusing on future ages and stages. How will you remind yourself to stay focused on the present age so you can help yourself and your child build skills to expand on in future stages?

- Consider how you will apply the information in this chapter to help you develop a relaxed readiness approach to allergy management and be mindful of all the important developmental processes. What specific actions and thoughts would help you do this?
- Add topics from this chapter to your growing list of allergy-related fears, worries, and questions to discuss with your child's allergist.

CHAPTER 4

Responding Differently to Anxious Thoughts

Jasmine came to therapy 6 months after her 14-year-old daughter had experienced anaphylaxis when she accidentally ate a cookie that contained peanuts while hanging out at a friend's house. After her daughter's peanut allergy diagnosis at nine months old, Jasmine had adjusted to allergy parenting and developed a workable balance between being cautious and letting her daughter live life fully—that is, until her daughter's most recent reaction. Jasmine knew that an increased feeling of anxiety and overwhelm after an allergic reaction was normal and expected, but six months later, she still found that her anxious thoughts were impacting her daily functioning and pushing her to continue restricting her daughter's social experiences beyond what was necessary. No matter what she tried and despite her daughter having safely navigated several social outings since the reaction, her mind kept focusing on anaphylaxis, convincing her that unless she kept her daughter home all the time, it would lead to another reaction . . . or worse, a life-threatening one. Of course, this line of thinking and restricting her daughter's activities outside of the house caused conflict between Jasmine and her daughter. Because of this, Jasmine knew it was time for her to reach out to an allergy-informed therapist to learn how to regain a balanced, relaxed readiness approach to her daughter's food allergy so that it didn't continue impacting her daily functioning and her daughter's social and developmental health.

Jasmine's daughter's most recent reaction led her to think the worst—thoughts like *Allergic reactions will always lead to death*, and *My daughter is safe only when she's home*—which led Jasmine to try controlling everything in her daughter's life. She was stuck in an overwhelmingly uncomfortable headspace and wished she could turn these thoughts off. Like Jasmine, I'm sure we all wish we had a delete button in our brain that would erase uncomfortable thoughts as soon as they pop into our awareness. Unfortunately, since no such thing exists, and because minds will do what minds do—think—we are forced to make choices about how to respond to and interact with our thoughts. What's more, the mind is complex and can entertain many thoughts at once—even ones that are seemingly opposite, such as *I can't deal with this* and *I've got to figure out how to handle this*. While our mind's ability to generate many thoughts at once can be useful, it also easily gives way to confusion, self-doubt, and overwhelm when making choices. I often tell my clients that the mind can be a dangerous neighborhood to get stuck in alone because it's filled with lurking thoughts just waiting to push you toward feelings you may not want to experience and actions that don't align with your values and goals. If we were to peek inside the mind of an allergy parent, you'd see a neighborhood filled with lots of dark corners harboring fear-based thoughts, second-guessing, and confusion about how best to navigate allergy life. It's also important to know that your mind often engages in a negativity bias, which means that it weighs negative experiences more heavily than it does positive ones, which in turn can lead you to make decisions based on negative information rather than on positive data.[1] Essentially, we have evolved to be on the lookout for anything that could threaten our survival. That's why your child's past allergic reactions or asthma attacks will be what your mind wants to dwell on—even if it has been years since they've happened, and you've had positive experiences since then. Together, all of this makes it hard to turn off anxiety autopilot and parent the way you want to.

Like Jasmine and many other allergy parents, you'll benefit from the mindfulness-based strategies discussed in this chapter, as they will help you respond differently to the anxiety-inducing, overwhelming thoughts you're experiencing on this allergy parenting journey—the ones that convince you that life with allergies is always scary and lead you to parent based on these anxious thoughts. Becoming more aware of your anxious thoughts so that you're able to choose *how* you want to respond to them is key to turning off anxiety autopilot in allergy parenting—and life in general. But before we jump into developing these skills, let's pause to learn more about anxiety and how it impacts your mind and body.

THE ANXIOUS MIND AND BODY

Anxiety may feel like the enemy, but it isn't—it is a normal emotion that every human experiences. Yes, it feels uncomfortable to be anxious, but when low to moderate levels of anxiety show up, it's typically not problematic—even if it sometimes feels like it is. As an allergy parent, though, you may find yourself wrestling with intense, persistent anxiety that feels hard to manage and begins to dictate your parenting decisions. Because there's no magic wand to wish anxiety away—and truthfully, we wouldn't want to—it's useful to understand what anxiety is and how it impacts your mind and body so that you can develop a new, more functional relationship with it.

Anxiety is an emotion that encourages you to look ahead and worry about future-focused situations rather than stay focused on the here and now. It can also push you to reconnect with painful memories from the past to help you avoid more pain in the future. As we covered in a previous chapter, the mind does this because it's trying to keep you (and your child) safe from danger and threats. You'll know anxiety is present when your mind jumps into the long, winding "what-if" rabbit hole of ruminating about every possible worst-case scenario. (*What if there's an allergic reaction? What if epinephrine or the inhaler doesn't relieve symptoms? What if my child has an allergic reaction on the plane?*) If we were to look inside an anxious mind, we would probably observe a flurry of thoughts that looked very similar to the swirling snow in a freshly shaken snow globe. When we live with allergies, these swirling anxious thoughts are typically worries related to being exposed to allergens, having allergic reactions and asthma attacks, getting sick, eating out, traveling, and specific phobias, such as needle phobia.[2]

Because anxiety brings with it overwhelming, racing thoughts, it's often labeled as a negative or bad emotion. So, does it surprise you that anxiety can also be helpful? At manageable levels, anxiety helps motivate us to plan, prepare, seek safety, and take meaningful actions. For instance, feeling anxious ahead of a job interview likely motivates you to practice your talking points so that you'll feel more confident during the interview. In allergy management, anxiety is useful because it helps you evaluate allergy-related risks, prepare safety plans, and problem-solve challenging and unsafe situations. But here's how anxiety goes from being helpful to being unhelpful, and even problematic. It's easy to assume that the mind's built-in threat scanner acts as a protective guide and that any anxious or fear-based thought you have is one you should follow to keep your child safe. Yet automatically believing anxious thoughts is risky, too, because a very anxious mind tends to distort things by encouraging you to overestimate risk and scary outcomes while also pushing you to underestimate your ability to navigate anxiety-inducing situations. Not a helpful combination of thoughts, right?

Remember, your mind does this because it's trying to motivate you to take actions that keep you and your child safe out in the world—and even safe from your own uncomfortable thoughts. Unfortunately, the mind often does its job too well and becomes unhelpful by convincing you that when something makes you feel anxious or uneasy, it must be unsafe. That then reinforces the unhelpful belief that things are safe only when you're not feeling anxious. But remember, anxiety is a normal emotion just like sadness and joy, so it's not possible to eliminate it. Therefore, equating allergy safety with being anxiety-free is misleading when assessing how safe an experience might be. All of this makes it harder for you to evaluate allergy-related risk levels and determine which risks are actual (real risks) and which ones are perceived (assumption or sense of risk). Next thing you know, the list of situations (and thoughts) you're trying to avoid becomes longer than the list of things you're willing to experience, because it feels easier—and safer—to avoid anything that makes you feel the least bit anxious about your child's safety.

For families managing food allergies, three key events tend to increase anxiety levels: (1) new accidental exposures, (2) new information regarding potential risks, and

(3) developmental transitions that threaten to increase exposure to risks.[3] Even in families who have been able to approach allergies with relaxed readiness, a new threat of danger can push them off course and back into a dysfunctional state filled with intense anxiety that impacts their ability to assess actual (real) risks versus perceived (assumed) risks. But safety concerns aren't the only times when anxiety and anxious thoughts show up. They also show up when you do something new, are unsure of an outcome, and when something is important to you. For example, I feel anxious when my oldest child flies a plane each weekend during his flight lessons. Yes, there are risks associated with flying planes, but I am also anxious because his flying is still new to us, I can't control if his flights will go safely, and because I love him. Therefore, it's appropriate for me to feel anxious when he's flying. But if I believed my unhelpful, overly anxious mind when it tried to convince me that I felt anxious only because flying was too unsafe (despite the long list of safety checks he performs and the data that show flying is safe), then I would automatically react by telling my son he couldn't do flight lessons and crush his dreams of becoming a pilot. Similarly, if I were to automatically let my anxious thoughts decide how I parented my food-allergic teenager, he would never leave the house, which would make his life miserable (not to mention negatively impact our relationship). Navigating flight lessons, allergy parenting, and other stressful situations in life has led me to develop a new relationship with my anxious thoughts—one that is built on the awareness of what happens when I feel anxious, the understanding that anxiety can be present for reasons beyond safety concerns, and that my choices and actions don't have to align with what my anxious mind says. As

you learn how to become more aware of your thoughts—especially the anxious ones—you'll be able to develop a new relationship with anxiety, too.

That brings us to the physical aspects of anxiety, and more specifically, fear. Have you ever observed what's happening within your body when you feel anxious and fearful? You've probably noticed the following bodily sensations when faced with danger or a threat to your child's safety: increased heart rate and blood pressure, clammy hands, upset stomach, tense or twitchy muscles, and heightened senses (to help you notice danger).[4] These bodily sensations and changes are part of the *fight or flight response* to stress. Once fear signals the danger alarm, our sympathetic nervous system responds with hormonal changes that physically prepare us to fight back or flee to safety. But here's the kicker: This stress response can overreact to stressors that aren't life-threatening. That means that your child doesn't have to be in actual danger or under threat for fight or flight to kick in; even anticipating or thinking about your child having an allergic reaction or asthma attack can turn it on. It's no surprise, then, that this further complicates the process of determining which allergy-related risks are actual and which ones are perceived. Given that you're constantly on high alert and scanning the world for allergy-related dangers, it's easy to perceive many things as threatening to your child's health and safety. Thus, fight or flight mode is never far away and can switch on at any moment, meaning your body might perpetually be stuck in that exhausting stress response cycle—which adds to the overwhelm in allergy parenting.

In addition to adding to the overwhelm of allergy parenting, it's worth noting that research tells us that chronic or long-term stress (resulting in chronic activation of the fight or flight stress response) can negatively impact our overall health.[5] Therefore, this is another area of allergy parenting that requires balance—helping your mind and body find balance between being *ready to act* and living in a state of *relaxed readiness* so that you're not perpetually in fight or flight mode and negatively impacting your own health. That's where your parasympathetic nervous system enters the picture. Whereas the sympathetic nervous system governs fight or flight mode, the parasympathetic nervous system governs *rest and digest mode*, which helps you relax and restore energy. When your body is in rest and digest mode, your heart rate and breathing decrease, and your bodily systems stabilize. The goal is for these two systems to work in harmony, finding a balance that allows you to respond to stress and then rest to restore energy. Unfortunately, sometimes these involuntary systems (which react to stressors on their own) don't work well together, and your body seems to constantly react to non-life-threatening stressors as if you or your child were in imminent danger.

While we can't control these systems, one way to help your body get back to rest and digest quicker after it goes into fight or flight is to practice deep breathing exercises.[6] When we feel anxious and stressed, we tend to take shallow breaths (also known as *chest breathing*) that don't fully engage both the chest and belly, which can lead to reduced oxygen intake and muscle tension. Alternatively, deep breathing (also known as *belly breathing*) encourages inhaling and exhaling slowly while engaging the diaphragm and belly as well as the chest so you experience a full oxygen exchange that helps the body stabilize. The simplest way to do this is to make sure that your belly

Pause and Practice: Square or Box Breathing

One easy way to perform belly breathing is to practice *square or box breathing*. Pause for a moment and practice this breathing technique so that you can feel the mind and body benefits.

To begin, think of a square or draw one on a piece of paper so you can use it as a guide while tracing it with your finger. With this square in mind or on your paper, do the following:

- As you trace across the top of the square, inhale for four seconds.
- As you trace down one side of the square, hold that breath for four seconds.
- As you trace across the bottom of the square, exhale for four seconds.
- As you trace up the other side of the square, hold (without inhaling) for four seconds.

Repeat this exercise a few times or as many times as you need until you feel calmer. If square or box breathing doesn't feel like a good fit, there are many other breathing exercises you can try. In the resource section at the back of this book, I've listed a variety of breathing exercises that offer calming benefits—all of which you can find video guides for online. The best part is that your whole family can learn how to calm their mind and body since many of these exercises can be taught to or adapted for children.

acts like a balloon—expanding when you inhale and deflating as you exhale.

Beyond breathing exercises, it's useful to begin noticing how your mind and body respond to potential threats to your child's health and safety. Pay attention to how frequently your anxious thoughts impact the perception that your child is in immediate danger, how your body responds in the face of those perceived threats, and what actions you take because of this interplay. Practice using calming breaths to help your body switch back to rest and digest mode so that your mind can respond to anxious thoughts without the intense sense of urgency. All of this will help you work toward accurately assessing allergy-related risks and approaching allergies with relaxed readiness.

After learning so much about anxiety, you may find yourself wondering when it's time to reach out for mental health services for yourself and/or your child, especially if you're noticing an ongoing elevated level of anxiety. In general, it may be time to consider therapy when you notice that your own or your child's thoughts, feelings, or actions are moderately or significantly impacting normal daily functioning, especially if that has been the case for an extended period. Psychologist Linda Herbert and her colleagues suggest that therapy might be useful for allergy families when you or your child already has a diagnosable mental health disorder or when there's difficulty coping with allergy-related anxiety, worries about allergic reactions are ongoing, and there are challenges in transitioning allergy management to the child or adolescent.[7] If you're unsure how to locate a therapist in your area, allergy-informed or otherwise, you'll find a list of therapist directories in the resource section at the back of this book.

In addition, it's worth noting that it's common (and understandable) to experience increased anxiety when considering oral food challenges and food allergy treatments (e.g., oral and sublingual immunotherapy). Anxiety about these processes commonly stems from (1) not knowing what to expect during these processes, (2) fears about potential allergic reactions, and (3) not knowing how allergic reactions will be addressed during these appointments. Talking with an allergy-informed therapist can be useful to address this anxiety, but often, simply talking with your child's allergist is helpful enough, especially since they may not realize fear is preventing you from pursuing these appointments. If your child's allergist is recommending oral food challenges and/or food allergy treatments, I encourage you to make an appointment to discuss related fears and to allow them an opportunity to present information to you about the benefits these processes have on quality of life and anxiety levels.

Finally, if you find yourself assuming that every situation is a high-risk threat to your child (and/or find yourself constantly in fight or flight mode), talk with your child's allergist to learn how to accurately determine allergy-related risk levels rather than letting your anxious mind determine them. To help you prepare for this conversation, refer back to the risk assessment and "safe enough" discussion in Chapter 2, which is located in the "Over-Avoidance Trap" section.

THE PROBLEM WITH TRYING TO AVOID OR CONTROL ANXIOUS THOUGHTS

When we initially began working together, Jasmine was in constant struggle with her anxious allergy-related thoughts. All she wanted to do was ignore her thoughts and the physical discomfort they brought when they convinced her that her daughter could no longer be safe at her friends' houses. Anytime she considered letting her daughter go out, she experienced a fight or flight stress response, which in her mind, reinforced her safety concerns and decisions to restrict her daughter's activities. Keeping her daughter home not only felt safer, but also helped Jasmine avoid the anxious thoughts and worry she'd have to deal with if she let her daughter go back to the place where her allergic reaction happened months earlier. Nevertheless, after noticing the negative impacts this approach had—leading her daughter to feel depressed and putting a strain on their relationship—Jasmine realized a change was needed. She needed to work toward developing the willingness to let her daughter hang out with her friends again, no matter how hard it would feel to do so.

Have you ever paid attention to what you do when engaged in a struggle with anxious thoughts? More specifically, have you noticed how much time and energy you use trying to control or distract yourself from anxious allergy-related thoughts? We all engage in behaviors that help us ignore, avoid, or control uncomfortable thoughts. Maybe you scroll through social media or, like me, mindlessly watch *Friends* for the thousandth time because it keeps you distracted. You might procrastinate calling your child's allergist to discuss something important because you want to keep your anxious thoughts at bay. Or maybe you play the "don't think about a pink elephant" game, constantly telling yourself not to pay attention to your anxious thoughts. Because we don't like experiencing discomfort—including uncomfortable thoughts and feelings—we often engage in *experiential avoidance*, meaning we engage in actions (like the ones I mentioned) that help us avoid, change, reduce, or eliminate uncomfortable thoughts, feelings, and sensations.[8] But to quote the infamous Dr. Phil, How's that working for you?

While it probably works for a bit, here are two reasons why trying to ignore, avoid, or control your anxious thoughts is problematic: (1) These attempts only work temporarily or in the short term, and (2) even when they do work, an emotional or experiential cost to you, your child, and your family is usually the result. The most common costs include feeling exhausted (from engaging in constant struggle and control battles with your thoughts), missing out on living in (and enjoying) the present moment, and not learning skills that help you (and your child) manage anxiety, which often leads to experiencing more anxiety in the long term. When allergy parents constantly try to avoid or control their anxious allergy thoughts, they often find themselves lacking the will (and energy) to adapt to life with allergies. That, in turn, hinders the ability to develop a relaxed readiness approach to allergy management, which ultimately comes at the expense of the child's emotional, social, and developmental well-being.

With all this in mind, I encourage allergy parents to consider the idea of workability. In ACT, assessing *workability* means evaluating whether your actions and choices are "working" in terms of effectively solving the problem, moving you toward your goals, and allowing you to live in alignment with your values.[9]

Pause and Practice: Assess the Workability of Trying to Ignore, Avoid, or Control Your Thoughts

The question "Is this workable for me and my family?" is often a pivot-point because it helps people recognize that a change of actions or how you manage thoughts and emotions may be needed, which is what Jasmine realized. To explore the workability of how you approach your thoughts, think of a recent time when an anxious allergy-related thought arose and answer the following questions:

- What was the thought?
- What did you do in response to the thought—did you try to ignore, avoid, or control it?
- In what ways did your approach help you temporarily feel better?
- In what ways did your approach result in emotional or experiential costs to you, your child, or your family?
- Are you willing to continue trying to ignore, avoid, or control your anxious allergy-related thoughts if doing so comes with these costs?

Therefore, even if avoiding and controlling your anxious allergy-related thoughts might "work" temporarily, does this approach feel *workable* for you and your family?

Now that we've established how anxiety impacts the mind and body, and how trying to ignore, avoid or control anxious thoughts often comes with emotional and experiential costs, let's explore strategies to help you respond to your anxious allergy-related thoughts in more useful, workable ways.

FOCUS ON THE PRESENT MOMENT TO STAY GROUNDED WHEN FEELING ANXIOUS

As soon as we began working together, I encouraged Jasmine to pay attention to where her mind was focused. In any given moment, I wanted Jasmine to determine if her mind was stuck in the past, grounded in the present, or focused on the future. Jasmine quickly realized that her mind was often focused on the painful memories about past allergic reactions, but this was for good reason. Jasmine's mind was acting as her protector, trying to help her (and her daughter) avoid feeling more pain, which future allergic reactions would surely bring. Unfortunately, this meant that Jasmine couldn't stay mindfully connected with the here and now.

Why is staying connected with the here and now so important? Because flexibly and purposefully remaining in the present moment by being mindful of your thoughts, feelings, sensations, and potential behaviors (even during distressing experiences) is a key component of being psychologically flexible, or being able to deal with whatever life throws your way. Since many of our thoughts, especially when anxious, are focused on past events or future worries, it becomes difficult to accurately observe what's happening in any given situation and therefore often leads to automatically *reacting* to challenges rather than *mindfully navigating* them. Yet, when you're connected with the present moment, you aren't overly focused on thoughts having to do with the past or future, so you are able to notice what's happening inside your mind and body so that you can mindfully make choices. Seems simple enough in theory, but it's hard to do until you begin paying attention to where your mind is focused.

Pause and Practice: Notice Where Your Mind is Focused

When living with allergies, it often feels as if life throws lots of challenges your way. Being able to stay grounded in the here and now and acknowledge whatever thoughts and feelings arise will help you more effectively navigate these challenges. Additionally, being able to stay present-focused is a skill that helps you respond more effectively to anxious thoughts, much like learning how to jump over hurdles rather than walking off the track when it feels challenging to reach the finish line.

Practice noticing if you're staying in the present moment by reflecting on where your mind has been focused while reading this book:

- Have you been able to stay in contact with the present moment and mindfully connect with what you're reading?
- Have you noticed that your mind has wanted to recall difficult past experiences, such as previous allergic reactions and asthma attacks?
- How often has your mind drifted off to focus on future worries about how to keep your child healthy and safe?

Any time you notice your mind continuing to wander away from the present moment—whether it's while reading the rest of this book or navigating a challenging situation—gently bring it back to the here and now by engaging your five senses. You can do this by noticing what you see, feel, hear, smell, and taste so that your mind can ground itself in the present moment again.

Go ahead and practice engaging your five senses right now. Observe what you see in the space around you, what your hands and feet are touching, what noises you can hear, what smells might be in the air, and if there's a particular taste in your mouth. Notice how doing this helps to bring your attention back to yourself and the space around you, which helps you pause from engaging with past- and future-focused thinking. Repeat this brief exercise as often as necessary when you notice your mind focusing on the past or future rather than on the present.

UNHOOK FROM YOUR ANXIOUS THOUGHTS

So far, we've established that the mind is a complex entity, that anxiety stirs up worry-focused thoughts that pull you out of the present moment, and that we often try to ignore, avoid, or control these anxious thoughts to decrease the discomfort we feel. Now, let's explore what to do when you become so tangled up in your anxious thoughts that you feel stuck and unable to move forward.

Imagine you're walking through a forest preserve not on a clear trail, but on a trail that is blocked by overgrown bushes and weeds. You know you need to keep moving forward to get back to your car, but it's hard to get anywhere because you keep getting tangled up in branches. You feel stuck and unsure how to proceed. This is what it feels like when you're experiencing *cognitive fusion*, which is a term in Acceptance and Commitment Therapy (ACT) that refers to becoming so tightly intertwined with your thoughts that you can't separate yourself from them, thereby taking these thoughts literally without noticing the process of thinking.[10] When this happens, it's as if you're experiencing tunnel vision—unable to focus on any other thoughts (other than the ones you're fused with), notice what's happening in the world around you, and envision a workable path forward.

Like experiential avoidance, cognitive fusion hinders your ability to be psychologically flexible or deal with whatever thoughts, feelings, or situations come your way. Instead, cognitive fusion pushes you to live by rigid, rule-governed thoughts and beliefs that lead you to excessively avoid situations in the name of safety, making your family's world feel smaller and more limited. These thoughts typically include words like "should" and "must" and tend to convince you that change is impossible, which leads to inflexible behaviors and actions. For instance, after her daughter's recent allergic reaction, the two unhelpful rule-governed thoughts that guided Jasmine's decisions were *Allergic reactions will always lead to death*, and *I must keep my daughter home because otherwise she won't be safe.* She became so fused with these rigid (and untrue) beliefs that they became her reality, skewing her perceptions and her decision-making. It also left her unable to consider more flexible, empowering thoughts such as *Allergic reactions don't always result in death*, and *If my daughter has another allergic reaction, we know how to respond*. She had convinced herself that they needed to live by these rigid beliefs for her daughter to stay safe and had become unwilling to consider any other paths forward. Yet, staying tangled up in these two thoughts left her perpetually stuck in a fearful, anxious state and unable to notice how this was impacting her daughter's emotional well-being—it was as if she was stuck and not able to see any other perspective.

When you're so tangled up in anxious allergy-related thoughts the way that Jasmine was, practicing *cognitive defusion* strategies helps you detach and untangle yourself from your thoughts so that you can see thoughts for what they are and make choices based on values rather than unhelpful thoughts.[11] This detaching is often referred to as *unhooking from your thoughts*, just like a fisherman detaches a fish (you) from a hook (your thoughts).

So, how do you engage in cognitive defusion? Try the following three strategies that were compiled by psychologists Elizabeth Gifford, Steve Hayes and Kirk Stroshal, all of whom helped establish ACT as a formal psychotherapy approach.[12]

Practice mental appreciation: Practicing mental appreciation starts by envisioning your mind as a separate part of you and then thanking it for the thoughts and feelings it produces. Remember that your mind offers up anxious and uncomfortable thoughts as a way to encourage you to pursue safety, even if it overshoots its goal and becomes unhelpful. Saying "Thank you mind for encouraging me to keep my child safe and healthy" helps you detach from the rigid, rule-governed thoughts that often become problematic.

Remember that thoughts are just thoughts: Reminding yourself that thoughts are ideas developed by your mind (aimed at helping you make sense of things) helps you unhook from them and keeps you from giving them too much power over you and your choices. Thoughts themselves do not cause negative outcomes or predict future experiences, but we often act as if they do. Instead, practice saying to yourself, "Is it possible to have that thought *and* do x, y, z?" For instance, "Is it possible to think that all family gatherings are unsafe *and* still be willing to have discussions with family members to explore how we can safely attend?" (The answer is yes, even if the outcome isn't always one that will allow you to attend safely.)

Say your thoughts out loud: Overwhelming and uncomfortable thoughts tend to swirl around in your mind, so saying them out loud allows you to explore them differently, helping you separate yourself from your thoughts. Try saying your thoughts slowly, making sure your mind isn't on autopilot so that you can really listen to the wordzs. You can even expand on this strategy by saying your thoughts in different voices or singing them.

MINDFULLY ACCEPT AND OBSERVE YOUR ANXIOUS THOUGHTS

When I talk with my clients about dealing with and unhooking from anxious allergy-related thoughts, the concept of acceptance quickly becomes part of the conversation. Most people often (wrongly) assume that when I encourage them to practice acceptance, I'm telling them that they must be okay with whatever thoughts, feelings, and urges they're experiencing. Yet in the ACT context, that's not what practicing acceptance means. Rather, *acceptance* means being aware of and mindfully observing your internal experiences (thoughts, feelings, memories, impulses) without automatically following them or trying to change them.[13]

Two major benefits of practicing acceptance with your thoughts are that (1) doing so helps you from trying to resist, avoid, and control your thoughts—which we've established isn't helpful and comes at a cost, and 2) doing so helps you create much-needed space between yourself and your thoughts, allowing you to explore them without judgment and then purposefully choose how you'd like to respond and proceed. All of this helps you become more psychologically flexible and understand that you aren't the thoughts and feelings you experience, but rather, you're an observer who mindfully notices them happening within you and can unhook from them.

Being a mindful observer of your thoughts and other inner experiences is like watching them on television as they happen in a movie scene. So, how do you become a mindful observer of your own thoughts? For starters, it requires getting out of autopilot mode—you know, the mode that you're in when you drive to the store without actively thinking about how to get there. Typically, you're on autopilot because you're too engaged in your thoughts and other internal experiences to pay mindful attention to what you're doing and what's going on around you. Unfortunately, your mind is usually busy with unhelpful, judgmental, anxiety-inducing thoughts when it's on autopilot since those are the types of thoughts the mind likes to default to.

To become an observer of your own thoughts, you must purposefully decide to switch autopilot off and pay attention to what's happening within your mind. (To help with this, I encourage you to visualize turning autopilot off by pushing a button, just as a pilot does when they turn off autopilot in a plane.) Once autopilot is off, use observing phrases like *I'm noticing the thought that . . .* and *I'm aware that my mind is saying . . .* as you observe the various thoughts that are popping up. Get curious and pay attention to various details. What are your thoughts saying about you, the world around you, and what it means to live with allergies? What tone do they have—judgmental or kind? Do they move through your mind easily, or do they stay stuck right in the forefront? Beyond just noticing the thoughts swirling around in your mind, it's also helpful to pay attention to how your thoughts impact you. How do they make your body feel? What other thoughts do they lead you to engage with? What emotions and memories do you notice rising to the surface of your mind while observing your thoughts? What actions do they lead you to take (such as experientially avoiding other thoughts and/or physically avoiding situations)? Accepting whatever comes up when thinking about parenting a child with allergies and taking this mindful, exploratory stance puts space between you and your thoughts, which allows you to observe how your mind moves from point A to point B (or Z). All of this is helpful when wanting to parent based on your goals and values rather than the overwhelming things your mind is telling you about parenting a child with allergies.

Because it can be hard to envision what it looks like to mindfully observe your thoughts without doing anything with them, consider the following analogies to help you as you work on developing this skill:

- Curiously observing your thoughts is like watching fish of all shapes and sizes in a pond. Imagine that from the edge of the pond (or your mind) you're observing your thoughts as if they were fish swimming around freely.

- Curiously noticing your thoughts is also like watching floats go by in a parade.[14] Imagine yourself watching your thoughts drive by in front of you as you notice various details about them, just as you do with colorful floats in a parade.
- Curiously watching your thoughts can also be like watching clouds in the sky. Become a "cloud gazer" with your thoughts, observing how they form and change as they float around in your mind just as you do while watching the clouds in the sky.[15]

To help further illustrate mindfully observing thoughts, here's an example focused on anxious allergy-related thoughts about traveling with food allergies: *I'm noticing thoughts about our upcoming trip. I'm aware that these thoughts make me feel anxious because they're focused on everything that could go wrong. Now I notice that I'm remembering how scary it felt when my child had an allergic reaction and how I don't want to feel that way ever again. I'm now observing that I feel nauseous and am thinking we should just cancel the trip.* Did you notice the use of observer phrases and how that helped to see how one thought led to another? Now it's your turn to practice.

Pause and Practice: Become a Mindful Observer of Your Thoughts

Let's practice how to mindfully observe a thought so you can use this skill to help you unhook from anxious ones. Normally, I'd encourage you to be aware of all the thoughts swirling around in your mind (like the snow in

(*continued*)

the snow globe), but it's easiest to practice with one specific thought when you're developing this skill. So choose one thought you notice running through your mind right now. It doesn't have to be related to allergies—it can be about anything. (*For example, the thought I'm focusing on right now is "I hope readers find this book helpful."*)

First, notice if the thought itself is pleasant, unpleasant, or neutral in tone. (*My initial thought is pleasant because it's focused on helping people.*) Is it judgmental or kind? (*My thought has a tone of self-judgment because I worry that my words won't help others.*) Does the thought feel heavy and sticky, like it wants to hang around in your mind for a while, or does it feel light, like it could come and go easily? (*My thought feels heavy and sticky—like it might stick around forever.*) Is the thought pulling you into past experiences, pushing you to focus on future worries, or helping you to engage in the current moment? (*My thought is future-focused, which is pulling me away from focusing on what I'm doing in the here and now.*) Next, check in with your body as you explore this thought and notice if you're feeling any physical sensations, such as tension, hunched shoulders, shallow breathing, or an upset stomach. (*Since I'm now feeling stressed about whether this book will be helpful, I'm noticing I am hunching my shoulders and feeling tension as I sit here at my computer.*) Then, notice whether the thought is stirring up emotions that might make you want to react to the thought by trying to control or avoid it all together.

(*This thought has stirred up anxiety, which makes me want to avoid it altogether by shutting my laptop and scrolling on social media instead.*) The thought might also lead to a bunch of additional thoughts or even encourage your mind to create a whole story about it. (*Yep! My mind has now created an unhelpful story about how my writing skills are bad and that this book won't help people, all of which came from that initial thought that I hope readers find this book helpful.*)

It's okay if mindfully observing a thought feels hard to do—that's normal and it will get easier with practice.

Like many allergy parents do, Jasmine initially struggled with the idea of accepting that she might always have anxious thoughts about her daughter's safety. However, her mindset started shifting after learning to mindfully notice her anxious thoughts and allow them to be there without needing to act on them, control them, or avoid them. At first, being a mindful observer of her thoughts felt hard, very unnatural, and even uncomfortable—all of which is normal because developing a new emotional wellness skill is like learning a new language. But after continued practice, Jasmine found that the space that she created between herself and her anxious allergy-related thoughts led to her experiencing fewer urges to control and avoid them, which also helped her feel less hooked by them. Yes, she still felt anxious when thinking about letting her daughter go to a friend's house, but being mindfully aware of her thoughts allowed her to talk herself through the anxiety so that she could consider other thoughts, choices, and outcomes.

Are you curious if Jasmine was able to get back to a relaxed readiness approach to her daughter's food allergy after working together? I'm happy to report that she was. Jasmine said that learning why her mind was anxious and that being anxiety-free wasn't the goal (and also didn't determine allergy-related safety) helped her develop the willingness to practice mindfully observing and unhooking from her anxious allergy-related thoughts. She began taking baby steps toward letting her daughter hang out at friends' houses again, slowly building up confidence in her daughter's ability to stay safe and effectively respond to emergencies if needed. Jasmine said that learning how to respond to her anxious allergy-related thoughts differently was pivotal in helping her work back to a relaxed readiness approach to allergy management (rather than continuing to parent on anxiety autopilot), and of course, it helped her relationship with her daughter, too.

TAKEAWAYS

- Allergy-related anxious thoughts often complicate your ability to evaluate allergy-related risks. They also make it harder to make parenting choices that are based on what's important and workable for your family.
- It can feel uncomfortable to mindfully observe anxious thoughts (allergy-related or otherwise), but trying to ignore, avoid, or control them typically causes more anxiety and often comes at an emotional and experiential cost.
- Aim to accept, mindfully observe, and unhook from your anxious allergy-related thoughts so that you can

approach allergy management with relaxed readiness and parent your child the way you want to, not the way your anxious thoughts dictate.

Think About and Do

- How have you been managing your anxious allergy-related thoughts up until now, and has that worked well for you?
- In what ways do your anxious allergy-related thoughts keep you from parenting the way you want to?
- Even though it might feel hard to do so, are you willing to practice the strategies shared in this chapter to develop a more workable approach to your anxious allergy-related thoughts? How might you start? Which strategies will you try first?

CHAPTER 5

Focusing on All That Matters—Not Just Allergy Safety

Tracy reached out to begin therapy after noticing increased conflict between her and her husband. They didn't see eye to eye about how they wanted to navigate life with food allergies, particularly when it came to traveling. Despite Tracy's having been an avid traveler prior to becoming a parent, parenting two children who managed multiple food allergies and asthma made travel feel too daunting for her. As a result, the family stopped traveling—even by car. Yet, if Tracy had been asked prior to these diagnoses how much of a role she thought travel would play in her family, she would have said it would play a huge role. In fact, Tracy had envisioned that she and her husband would be camping, backpacking, and traveling all over the world with their children because of their shared passion for travel and their desire to continue making it a priority. That all changed once the children were diagnosed with allergies.

In one of our sessions, I asked Tracy to imagine there was a magic wand that would allow her family to safely navigate the world with allergies. They wouldn't have to worry about anaphylaxis or asthma attacks or navigate painful thoughts about past reactions—they could just enjoy life without any restrictions. I asked Tracy to answer the following questions:

- How would you act differently as an allergy parent?
- What would you start doing, stop doing, and do more or less of?
- What experiences would you want your family to have that you've been afraid to pursue?
- What qualities would you want to focus on and encourage your children to develop beyond safety?

Here's how Tracy responded to these questions:

> If this magic wand helped us navigate life with allergies safely, I would act more spontaneously and flexibly. I would encourage my kids to be brave and adventurous and to seek out all sorts of experiences in their lives. As a family, we would make travel a priority by putting together a list of places we'd like to visit and check them off as we go. We would be making memories together.

For many allergy parents, anxiety, fear, and overwhelm get in the way of pursuing meaningful life experiences and living the way they want to live. Remember, though, that allergy parenting isn't made easier by trying to control or avoid your thoughts and feelings—and in fact, doing so makes it feel harder. Instead, your goal is to focus on living a full and meaningful life even with anxiety, fear, and a sense of overwhelm being present.

This chapter will introduce you to another tool that will help you realign with *all* that matters to your family so that you can work towards a more balanced, relaxed readiness approach to allergy management and so you don't feel as if allergies are keeping your family from living a full and meaningful life.

The magic wand scenario and the questions I asked above will begin to help you to identify what matters to you in life—beyond your child's health and safety. These are likely ways of living and important qualities that you may have lost touch with after becoming an allergy parent. Therefore, before you keep reading, pause for a moment to think about how you would answer the questions I asked Tracy.

WHAT VALUES ARE . . . AND ARE NOT

In previous chapters, we've explored unhelpful mindsets, the benefits of identifying allergy parenting traps and accurately assessing allergy-related risks, the importance of understanding developmentally focused parenting goals, and the usefulness of responding to anxious allergy-related thoughts differently. But there are more ingredients in the recipe for developing a mindful approach to allergy parenting and a relaxed readiness approach to allergy management, two of which we will explore in this chapter: *values* and *committed action*.

Let's start with values. While anxious allergy thoughts like to dictate how you *should* parent (often driven by unhelpful and rigid beliefs), values help you choose how you *want to* parent. In Acceptance and Commitment Therapy (ACT), values reflect what you find meaningful and important and guide your actions and ways of living.[1] They help you to behave in ways that align with who you want to be and help you to make purposeful choices even when you're responding to stressful experiences happening in any given moment.[2] They also give your life meaning and a sense of purpose as you navigate the world.

Essentially, values act as your compass helping to guide your directions in life, which is why I like to refer to values as your "North Stars." They are like GPS coordinates that you can refer back to when your anxious thoughts push you off the road as you travel to your destination—namely, raising a self-sufficient young adult who can independently manage their allergic condition.

Common values include, but certainly aren't limited to

- accountability
- achievement
- adaptability
- adventure
- assertiveness
- balance
- bravery
- connection
- cooperation
- courtesy
- courage
- creativity
- curiosity
- engagement
- exploration
- flexibility
- freedom
- grace
- gratitude

- honesty
- humility
- kindness
- independence
- integrity
- mindfulness
- patience
- persistence
- presence
- reliability
- respect/self-respect
- responsibility
- safety
- supportiveness
- travel
- trust
- vitality

To help solidify your understanding of values, let's briefly look at what values are not.

Values are not the same as goals, although people often confuse them. Goals are outcomes with definitive end points; they are tasks you can check off a list once you've accomplished them.[3] Sometimes goals can even be emotional in nature, such as having a goal to feel less or more of an emotion. Your values can help you achieve your goals. For instance, if your goal is to raise a child who can confidently manage their allergies while living independently, your parenting choices while in pursuit of these goals could be guided by empowering values such as courage, independence, and responsibility.

Values are not feelings either. Yes, you'd probably rather feel calm than anxious, but feelings aren't something we get to decide or control. In fact, just as with thoughts, the more we try to control feelings, the deeper we get into struggle with them. Instead, you get to choose how you'd like to respond to your feelings, using your values as a guide, especially if you've set an emotional goal such as wanting to feel less anxious. For example, when anxiety shows up, you can use your values (such as courage, patience, and supportiveness) to mindfully respond to your thoughts and bravely pursue meaningful actions even when anxious thoughts are present, which feels incredibly empowering.

Values are also not focused on others' choices and how you want to be treated by others. As an allergy parent, you want nothing more than for people to respect you, your child, and the allergy safety protocols you've put in place. Unfortunately, you don't have any control over how others treat you (or respect your allergy protocols). What *is* within your power is to embody your own value of respect, acting respectfully toward others, which may encourage them to show the same respect toward you—but that's their choice, not yours.

When Tracy identified which values were guiding her allergy parenting approaches, her main value was safety, as yours might be, too. Yet, when we explored what other values beyond safety were important to Tracy—ones she had likely been overlooking and not acting on—they included adaptability, adventure, courage, curiosity, exploration, flexibility, responsibility, and travel. These values had helped her become an avid traveler, yet she stopped prioritizing them after her children were diagnosed in service of prioritizing their safety.

Before we started working together, she hadn't realized that she had abandoned these important values. But as she learned—and you will too as you keep reading—we can simultaneously hold multiple values and make choices about how to balance and prioritize them rather than only holding one value. In fact, your life (and your child's life) will benefit from doing so.

Would you be able to identify your North Stars, or the values guiding your allergy parenting choices? It's understandable if you're struggling to define your values as you're reading this chapter. I admit that I struggled to draft a list of values when I first became an allergy parent, too. Use the "Pause and Reflect" exercise to help you begin drafting your values lists.

PAUSE AND REFLECT: CLARIFYING YOUR VALUES

One way to start identifying your values is by paying attention to how vulnerable or uncomfortable you feel in various experiences, as it is a good way to evaluate how much something matters to you.[4] As my friend Jill Stoddard, says, "What we fear is what we hold most dear." For instance, the thought of your child having an allergic reaction or asthma attack likely terrifies you, which makes sense. Therefore, it's safe to say that two values that are important to you are *safety* and *protection*. Since those two values are a given when parenting a child with allergies, my goal in this chapter is for you to explore other values that are important to you in addition to these two—and ones that you might be overlooking due to the overwhelm.

Another way to identify what values are important to you is by reflecting on others you admire. In her book *Be Mighty*, Jill encourages readers to explore their values by recalling a favorite person or character whom they admire, who possesses qualities that matter to them, or who inspires them.[5]

Since we're focusing on living with allergies, I'd like you to think of a person who lives with allergies or parents a child with allergies. You don't have to personally know them; maybe it's a parent within your community who has been managing allergies for years, an allergy advocate you're following online, or an allergy support group leader. (If you can't identify a specific person, perhaps because you don't know others managing allergies, think about an ideal allergy parent you'd likely admire and the qualities they'd possess.) Now, think about why you chose that person or ideal person. What do you admire about the way in which this person navigates life with allergies? What actions, choices, and personal qualities do they embody that make you think, "I'd like to act/behave/live like that!" How do they approach challenging situations, even ones that may initially feel daunting and unsafe? Focus on these things to help you draft your list of allergy parenting values. For instance, the person may choose to live courageously by pursuing travel despite feeling anxious about doing so. Or maybe the person is assertive about their allergy safety, speaking up and self-advocating in a way that is firm, yet kind and effective in educating others.

When I first became an allergy parent, I admired a mom whose child was 10 years older than my son. While I didn't know her well, the few conversations I had with her made an impact. She had developed a workable balance between safety and flexibility—adapting to her son's diagnosis and taking a relaxed readiness approach to life with food allergies despite the allergy anxiety she felt. Finding that balance was something I hoped to be able to do as well. She had also become an advocate for her son's health care, and as such, researched and found an allergist who would take a personalized approach to food allergy diagnosis (something that wasn't common in 2012 but is nowadays). She felt hopeful that her son could live a full and fun life *and* stay safe, too. Observing these qualities and how they guided her choices in allergy parenting was pivotal to my own perception of what kind of allergy parent I wanted to be. This was especially important because my son's initial food allergy test results were inconclusive about possible tree nut allergies in addition to his peanut allergy. Of course, this lack of clarity further fueled my allergy anxiety. Confused by this information and empowered by this mom's ability to advocate and develop a balanced approach to life with food allergies, I reached out to a different allergist and asked if they could help us get more accurate information. After repeating the allergy tests and doing tree nut oral food challenges, we learned that my son wasn't allergic to tree nuts and that it would be beneficial to incorporate them into his diet, which he still safely does to this day. Admiring this mom's approach to food allergy management helped me clarify my own values, which include adaptability, bravery, empowerment, optimism, and resilience. This, of course, set me on a different allergy parenting path than if I had stayed on the anxiety autopilot path—and that's my hope for you, too, as you clarify all of your allergy parenting values.

Reflecting on the person you admire and the sample values list from the previous section, I'd like you to jot down two sets of values:

- **Your parenting values:** Which values are important to you as an allergy parent? What kind of allergy parent do you want to be? What do you want to stand for? How do you want to show up in various allergy-related scenarios? This might include being adaptable when navigating challenging situations, choosing empowering actions, persevering when allergy parenting feels tough, leaning into gratitude more often, and speaking up about your child's allergy management needs even when it feels daunting doing so.

- **Your family's values:** What values do you want your child and your family to learn and live by? This might include wanting to cultivate bravery and courage, especially when outcomes are unknown. It may also include modeling the willingness to persevere through challenges to have fun and important experiences.

Remember, the value of safety (and wanting to be the protector) will always be a priority value, but for this exercise, I want you to think of the other values you want to focus on in addition to safety—ones that will help you approach allergy parenting and life in general in a more balanced manner.

WHY FOCUSING ONLY ON THE VALUE OF SAFETY CAN BE PROBLEMATIC

We've already established that safety is a value that will always be a priority when parenting a child with allergies. Under the circumstances, it's easy to rigidly define safety as "all or nothing" and believe that allowing for any amount of risk and uncertainty means that all safety is lost. Nevertheless, I will continue to highly encourage you to discuss allergy-related risks and safety in depth with your allergist to help you (1) clearly understand what they define as safe, safe enough, and not safe; (2) learn how to effectively evaluate allergy-related risks; and (3) clarify what actions are needed (and not needed) to ensure your child's safety. Gaining clarity on what allergy-related safety looks like and understanding the varying degrees of allergy-related risks will help you feel more willing to try living in alignment with multiple values. (To help you with this, refer back to the "Over-Avoidance Trap" section in Chapter 2 for the list of risk assessment conversations to have with your allergist.)

With all that said, what I am suggesting in this chapter is that safety becomes *one* of the values you focus on, not the *only* value you focus on. Why? Because focusing *only* on allergy safety—and more specifically, the rigid definition that safety is all or nothing—often comes at a cost. Even so, that pull to focus only on safety is strong for all parents, but especially allergy parents—it's like a supercharged magnet, pulling you toward it. Therefore, you'll have to mindfully choose to pursue balance between safety and other important values, even if it feels scary to do so.

To help motivate you to do this, let's explore why focusing only on the value of safety can perpetuate anxiety, intensify the overwhelm when parenting a child with allergies, and make it harder to be the allergy parent you want to be.

It Can Lead to Values Conflicts and Imbalances

Focusing only on safety values (because you believe focusing on anything else won't keep your child safe) opens the door to many values conflicts and imbalances in addition to perpetuating unhelpful anxious beliefs. Values conflicts and imbalances are exactly what they sound like—conflict and incompatibility between two or more of the values that are important to you and your family and the inability to find workable ways to engage with multiple values simultaneously. This often leads to a disconnection with other prioritized values (in service of focusing only on safety), which results in not living the way you want to, not doing the things that you enjoy, and avoiding life-enhancing experiences—beyond what is necessary—to stay safe. On top of that, the stress of these conflicts and imbalances can also negatively impact relationships with family and friends, leaving you feeling more isolated and alone in your allergy parenting journey.

Tracy clearly had a values imbalance when we first started working together, as she focused only on safety and dismissed all the other values that had previously been important to her. Additionally, she and her husband were engaged in a values conflict given they couldn't agree on how to approach life with allergies: He wanted to balance safety and adventure, while she wanted to focus only on safety.

So, what can you do when caught in values conflicts, internally or with a loved one, or when you notice values imbalances? The goal is to develop a workable balance between keeping your child safe and living in alignment with other values that are also important to your family. We'll explore a specific strategy to help you work toward this in just a moment.

It Can Reinforce Unhelpful Approaches to Anxious Allergy-Related Thoughts

Focusing only on the value of safety often leads you to engage with your anxious allergy thoughts in unhelpful ways (rather than helping you manage them), which keeps you from being psychologically flexible, or riding the waves of life as they come.

If you've been focused only on the value of safety, you've likely convinced yourself that safety is all or nothing and that doing anything that feels less than perfectly safe is literally dangerous to your child's health. If so, you'll continue to be hooked by the shoulds, musts, and have-tos, which means living life by rigid rules and beliefs that are often developed by your anxious mind. Living like this—psychologically inflexibly—makes it much harder to develop a relaxed readiness approach to allergy management and to simultaneously nurture your child's development, your own parental development, and the development of how you'll approach life with allergies. While we covered this in depth in the previous chapter, it's important to mention that focusing only on allergy safety (to the exclusion of other important values) actually perpetuates psychological inflexibility.

So, what can you do if solely focusing on safety is leading you to engage in unhelpful actions aimed at managing your anxious thoughts through control-seeking behaviors? Revisit the previous chapter to reinforce and practice the strategies discussed as you work toward approaching your anxious thoughts in more useful and workable ways.

It Can Negatively Impact Your Child's Overall Well-Being

As we've discussed throughout this book, how you approach allergy management has the potential to positively or negatively impact your child's overall well-being.

When parents focus only on the value of safety, it tends to be because they haven't yet learned effective ways to manage their anxious allergy thoughts, and instead, they let those thoughts dictate that safety is the only value that matters. This can lead parents into one or more of the allergy parenting traps we explored in Chapter 2, which makes it harder for them to develop a workable balance between the three developmental processes we explored in Chapter 3 (child development, parental development, and allergy management development). In addition, focusing solely on safety has the potential not only to teach the child that living with allergies requires that they do so as well (rather than holding multiple values), but also to impede their ability to meet normal childhood milestones and develop self-efficacy skills, as well as having negative impacts on their emotional and social health.

So, what can you do to help yourself stay aware of the pull to focus solely on the value of safety? Start by staying mindful of how doing so can impact your child's overall well-being. Also, check in with your parenting actions and choices, determining if their purpose is to relieve your own allergy anxiety or if they're in service of teaching your child how to effectively navigate life with allergies. The goal is to base your actions and choices on the latter, while also keeping your child safe and teaching them how to keep themselves safe, too.

Pause and Practice: Shift to an *AND* Mindset to Balance Safety and Other Values

When an allergy parent chooses to focus only on the value of safety, I describe this as living with an ***OR*** mindset, which perpetuates rigid and anxious thoughts, rather than an ***AND*** mindset, which encourages flexible thinking and the ability to prioritize multiple values.

Shifting to a more flexible ***AND*** mindset can feel hard, and even scary. It will require you to face your anxious allergy-related thoughts head on, but remember that in doing so, you're that much closer to turning off anxiety autopilot and being the allergy parent (and family) you envision being.

To help you begin to make this mindset shift, work through this exercise, repeating it any time you feel stuck

(*continued*)

in an ***OR*** mindset. I'm encouraging you to do this on paper initially, as it will feel helpful to visually see your thoughts in writing, but you can do this exercise in your mind once you get the hang of it. (See Tracy's example in Table 5.1, which can help illustrate this exercise.)

- First, make a chart with four columns.
- Label the first column *or*, the second column *and*, the third column *scenario*, and the fourth column *what*.
- In the first column, write your first *or* values statement, which likely has the word "should" or "must" in it (e.g., *We should focus on safety* or *connection*).
- In the second column, write your *and* values statement, which is more flexible and allows you to focus on more than one value (e.g., *We can focus on safety* and *connection*).
- In the third column write a scenario or life domain for which you'd like to use the ***AND*** mindset approach (e.g., balancing safety and another value while eating in restaurants).
- In the fourth column, write down what would help you focus on both values in that scenario. This might include
    - noticing when your mind pushes you towards rigid thinking
    - addressing your anxious allergy-related thoughts with your allergist
    - clarifying perceived versus actual allergy-related risks with your allergist
    - gathering more information from your allergist on how to navigate situations safely

- practicing stress management strategies like deep breathing
- eliminating the use of anxiety-inducing online information sources.

Table 5.1 Example of Tracy's *AND* Mindset Exercise

Scenario	*Or* Mindset	*And* Mindset	What Will Help
Traveling as a family	We must focus on safety ***or*** adventure.	We can be both safe ***and*** adventurous.	• Remember that I want to teach my children to be adventurous while staying safe. • Clarify actual versus perceived allergy-related risks related to traveling. • Consider places that don't feel as challenging to visit for the first couple of trips, to help build confidence.
Traveling options	We must focus on safety ***or*** flexibility.	We can be both safe ***and*** flexible.	• Notice unhelpful anxious thoughts and unhook from them. • Research allergens in areas we want to travel. • Discuss with allergist overall strategies for staying safe while traveling and specific strategies for the mode of transportation (e.g., airplane, car, train). • Based on discussions with allergist and risk-related comfort levels, consider traveling by car rather than by air.

(continued)

Repeat this process, pairing safety with other values from your values list and working through various scenarios and domains in which you find it hard to focus on anything beyond just allergy safety. As you continue to do this, you'll find it easier to lean into an ***AND*** mindset instead of an ***OR*** mindset.

LIVING BY YOUR VALUES MEANS ENGAGING IN COMMITTED ACTIONS

As we've established, your values are another tool to help guide you through the overwhelm of allergy parenting, in addition to developmentally focused allergy parenting goals. Both serve as compasses, keeping you on course and working toward all that matters. But identifying your allergy parenting values is only the first part of focusing on all that matters; the second part is engaging in *committed action.*

Simply stated, *committed action* involves engaging in values-aligned behaviors.[6] It involves practicing willingness, or choosing to make behavior changes in service of your values, and committing to taking those actions (even when doing so is hard) for the purpose of moving in the direction in which your values point you.[7] Whereas your values are the trail map and compass for your hike through life, committed actions are the steps you physically take as you walk along the hiking path.[8]

Here are a few examples of pursuing committed action in allergy parenting:

- tapping into courage as you introduce allergens and new foods to your child

- building the willingness to trust others to care for your child after educating them on your allergy management protocols
- encouraging responsibility in your child by teaching them how to carry their emergency medications and action plans
- cultivating creativity and flexibility by exploring (with your child's input) ways to safely navigate new experiences and activities that are important to them
- practicing patience with your co-parent as they learn all the allergy management information and strategies you already know so well.

Engaging in committed actions relating to the value of allergy-related safety is easy—you are already willing to choose actions aligned with protecting your child from allergic reactions and asthma attacks. But choosing to engage in actions aligned with your other values will likely feel much harder because it requires you to step outside of your comfort zone. This is especially true if you believe your unhelpful anxious mind when it tells you that you can't focus on anything other than your child's safety (otherwise bad things will happen). So it's going to take practice for you to become more comfortable acting in service of multiple values. Think of it like learning a new language: You'll need to practice this new way of approaching life with allergies if you want to develop more balance and reconnect with a sense of vitality rather than stay on autopilot.

To help you engage in committed action more regularly, especially as you're just beginning to do so, consider these practices:

Create a values cheat sheet: Jot down your top three values from your allergy parenting and/or family values lists and keep them handy—on your phone, the bulletin board, or the fridge, wherever you'll see them regularly. Before engaging in actions, especially relating to situations that feel anxiety-inducing, review your values lists (which includes safety and other values) and consider how you can act in service of all of them or at least two. Think about specific actions to take and how you might handle the anxious thoughts and physical sensations that will arise when doing something outside of your comfort zone.

Practice willingness: If it helps ease you into taking committed action, initially practice the willingness to act on your values outside of the allergy parenting domain. Choose another domain in your life (for instance, work or social), and choose one specific value to act on for one week at a time. Maybe you'll choose to focus on gratitude and giving thanks to co-workers when they've been helpful. Or you might focus on assertiveness and speak up when the date for your next get-together with friends doesn't work for you. Then work on transitioning these willingness practices to focus on taking values-aligned actions in allergy parenting.

Develop a family mantra: Using your family values list, choose one or more value. Use it to help your family develop a mantra, or a guiding statement that reminds you of what's important to your family. For example, if you choose courage, your mantra might be "Courage is taking brave leaps even when it feels hard to do so." As a family, you can discuss how this meaningful mantra can be used to help you engage in strategies that balance staying safe and living a life filled with fun experiences even while managing allergies.

Carry helpful reminders: Like the values cheat sheet, objects can remind you of your chosen values and the importance of living in alignment with them. For example, while visiting my in-laws last summer, I took a trip to the local cathedral and bought a little stone that says "believe" on it. I chose this stone because the word "believe" reminds me to live in alignment with my values when it feels hard to do so—especially when my anxious mind tries to convince me that encouraging my son to be adaptable, brave, flexible, and independent will lead to more allergic reactions. (That word "believe" is so important to me that I even have it tattooed on my inner wrist so that the reminder is always with me.) There will be plenty of things that might shake your willingness to take values-aligned committed action, so it can be incredibly helpful to have objects or reminders that encourage you to stay connected with all that matters, not just safety.

DOING WHAT MATTERS MOST, EVEN WHEN IT'S HARD

As I already mentioned, choosing to engage in actions that are aligned with other values beyond safety will likely feel hard at first. As I continued working to help Tracy take committed action aligned with the multiple values that she deemed important, barriers popped up that tried to push her off course. Specifically, these barriers were feelings of fear, pain, self-doubt, anxiety, and overwhelm. I reassured Tracy (often) that these feelings weren't signs that she was making unsafe choices; rather, they were feelings that reinforced Tracy's love for her children. Remember what my friend Jill says: "What we fear is what we hold most dear." She also aptly reminds us that living according to one's values also brings pain (and other uncomfortable feelings) *because* it's focused on who and what we care about.[9] In other words, you can expect to experience feelings of fear, pain, self-doubt, anxiety, and other uncomfortable emotions as you work toward taking committed action as an allergy parent, but that's because you love your child, not because you're making poor choices.

Therefore, when these feelings arise (and they will), you'll need to dig deep to remind yourself of the benefits you, your child, and your family will reap by taking values-aligned committed actions. These are your *whys*—reminders of why committed action, even when it feels hard to pursue, is worthwhile. Combining these whys with the desire to become the allergy parent and family you want to be (even with anxiety and overwhelm present) can help you stay motivated to continue pursuing meaningful actions in service of the overall well-being of your child, not just keeping them safe.

If in this process you find yourself getting hooked (cognitively fused) by unhelpful anxious allergy thoughts or you begin defaulting to excessive avoidance of life experiences and your own internal experiences (experiential avoidance), revisit and practice the cognitive defusion strategies shared in Chapter 4. In addition, consider whether there are unanswered questions and concerns getting in the way of pursuing these values—ones that you can address with your allergist—especially pertaining to perceived versus actual allergy-related risks in various situations. Also consider if there are allergy parenting traps you're still struggling to break free from, and if you're taking into consideration the allergy parenting goals for your child's current stage of development. Finally, consider flexible actions you can take to help you pursue committed action focused on multiple values, such as bringing your own food to social gatherings and renting a condo when traveling so you can cook meals. (We'll explore engaging in flexible behaviors in the next chapter.) All these things can be factors that influence your ability, and can become barriers, to living in alignment with all that matters to you, not just your child's safety and health.

Tracy kept saying how hard it felt to try living in alignment with multiple values, and I kept reminding her that "yes, this is hard, but also possible." Her determination to find a better balance between all the values she wanted her family to embody—not just safety—helped her persevere through the discomfort as she pursued many new committed actions. For instance, when she began researching travel destinations, she felt a mix of excitement and fear. While her anxious mind tried to convince her to stop, staying connected with her *whys*, which included wanting to teach her kids how to be both adventurous and safe, reminded her why pushing forward was worthwhile. She had already discussed her travel safety concerns with their allergist, and together, they developed strategies that helped Tracy feel as if traveling safely as a family was possible. She found that she needed to repeatedly unhook herself from her anxious thoughts and lean into her determination to truly work toward balancing all that mattered. And that's exactly what she did. Their first trip was to Disney World, which is well-known for accommodating allergies, but just a few road trips later, Tracy and her family flew across the country to visit family members they hadn't seen in years. Although anxious thoughts still popped up while planning and executing travel, and although there were bumps in the road at times, Tracy's hard work paid off, as she and the whole family were benefiting from focusing on all that mattered in addition to staying safe and healthy.

For Tracy and thousands of other allergy parents, including myself, it's possible to focus on keeping your child safe and healthy while also focusing on other aspects of life that matter to you. It just takes the willingness to take that first step in the direction of values-aligned living and the courage to pursue committed actions even when it feels hard (but is safe) to do so.

TAKEAWAYS

- Values are ways of living that are influenced by what you find meaningful and important, and they are another tool to help guide you through the overwhelm of allergy parenting.
- Simultaneously holding multiple values that you deem important (beyond the value of safety) will help you become the allergy parent you'd like to be and help your family incorporate meaningful experiences while managing allergies.
- Taking values-aligned committed actions involves choosing to make behavior changes even when doing so is hard.
- Staying connected to your *whys* and how you, your child, and your family will benefit from balancing all that's important will help you persevere when it feels

hard to act in service of multiple values that include, but don't only focus on, safety.

Think About and Do

- Choose one or two values from the values lists you created in this chapter and think about how life might look different by living in alignment with them—even when uncomfortable thoughts and feelings about allergies are present.
- Think about how it will feel for your family to engage in additional life experiences if you're willing to live in alignment with important values beyond just safety.
- Envision how you might feel as an allergy parent by embodying and modeling these important values and qualities for your child.

CHAPTER 6

Developing Flexible Perspectives on Allergy Parenting

As I was writing this book, the son who manages a peanut allergy experienced a major medical event (not allergy-related)—one that involved an ambulance, a hospital stay, and lots of tests. This medical event required us to learn about a new health diagnosis, make lifestyle adjustments, and explore possible treatment approaches, including a major surgery. Because he's a teenager and I respect his privacy, I won't share specifics, but I will share this: As a parent, adjusting to this new health condition felt similar to adjusting to his peanut allergy years earlier—completely overwhelming.

Here I was, a licensed therapist writing a book to help parents navigate the overwhelm of health diagnoses, yet I was struggling to emotionally stay afloat and maintain a workable perspective on my son's health. Once I realized that I had fallen back into anxiety autopilot after this medical event, I paused to observe how that was impacting my actions. What I noticed was that I had become hooked by my anxious thoughts about his health, had lost connection with many of my values (especially courage and flexibility), was using control-seeking behaviors to manage my anxiety, and had become excessively hypervigilant, constantly checking in on my son—not because I needed to, but because I was anxious. (I can't begin to tell you how annoyed he was with me.) I also noticed that I had become more critical and judgmental of myself since I felt ashamed for letting my anxious thoughts get the best of me even though I knew better. Yet, I didn't want to stay stuck in anxiety parenting mode and didn't want to limit my son's life because of my anxious thoughts about his health, so I guided myself back to mindful parenting—just as I did after his food allergy diagnosis. Through compassionate self-talk (*This is hard, so give yourself space and grace—you'll get there!*), mindfully noticing and responding to my anxious thoughts differently so I could unhook from them (*Thank you, mind, I know you're just trying to help*), and allowing multiple values to guide my actions (not just safety), I was able to turn anxiety autopilot off once again. This takes practice and effort, so if it doesn't come naturally to you at first, don't give up!

I'm sharing this story with you to illustrate a few things. First, life will keep life-ing, and life's ups and downs aren't something any of us has control over. That means that even after you've adjusted to life with allergies and have developed a workable, values-aligned approach to allergy management, something may happen to throw that balanced approach (and your perspective) into flux. Second, it's helpful to mindfully see yourself and your own actions as part of the world around you. Third, it's important to have tools and strategies, such as the ones I'm sharing in this book, to help you not only establish a workable approach to life with allergies, but also regain your balance and perspective when life throws you curveballs—because it will.

WHY PERSPECTIVE SHIFTING IS IMPORTANT IN ALLERGY PARENTING

Imagine that you have a piece of paper in front of you, and on that paper, I ask you to draw a timeline of the allergy parenting experiences you've had up until this point. Because of negativity bias and the mind being hardwired to seek safety over happiness, we tend to focus on negative experiences more than positive ones. So my guess is that you would default to writing down the anxiety-inducing moments, such as your child's diagnosis, allergic reactions, asthma attacks, and so on. Looking at a timeline filled with unpleasant events, what would your perspective on allergy parenting be? Probably negative and overwhelming.

But what if I asked you to add all the positive and neutral experiences you've had in allergy parenting to the timeline as well. This would include times when you navigated tough experiences successfully, when you observed your child exhibiting an understanding of their allergy, when you taught your child allergy management skills, when you found safe foods to eat, when you stayed safe while doing something outside of your comfort zone, and when you managed an allergic reaction well. If you were to look at your allergy parenting timeline with these added experiences, would you feel any different about allergy parenting than you did when looking at the timeline without them? My hope is that you'd have a more balanced perspective on your allergy parenting journey with a timeline that included a variety of experiences.

What I'm getting at in the example above is practicing *perspective shifting*. Perspective-shifting means being open-minded and willing to see situations from different angles and to consider multiple points of view. I like to describe perspective-shifting as widening your perspective from one that is tunnel-vision to one with panoramic views, allowing you to see a much fuller picture that includes multiple experiences and points of context. Taking a panoramic perspective (rather than a tunnel-vision perspective) offers a more balanced and flexible viewpoint rather than one that is inflexibly focused on negative experiences and unhelpful thoughts.

There are several benefits of practicing perspective shifting. For one thing, it encourages you to engage in a growth mindset (which we covered in Chapter 1) and allows you to reflect on your evolution as an allergy parent, to notice your allergy parenting wins, and to remind yourself that you're still learning new skills—all of which are useful when your mind gets stuck focusing on the struggles of allergy parenting. In fact, research shows that having the ability to adjust your viewpoint has positive impacts on marital satisfaction, parenting stress, and family alliance.[1] When living with ongoing health conditions, one's perspective on that condition can shift according to symptom management and impacts on daily functioning, with better managed conditions helping people to see their diagnosis as just one aspect of their lives, not the full focus.[2]

Finally, and perhaps most importantly, perspective shifting helps you become more *psychologically flexible*. As I mentioned earlier, navigating ongoing uncertainty and fear in allergy parenting makes it easy to become *psychologically inflexible*, which can lead you to getting hooked (cognitively fused) by anxious thoughts, engaging in experiential avoidance (or trying to avoid and control these uncomfortable thoughts), becoming disconnected from your chosen values (especially ones in addition to safety), and ultimately, making choices that lead to living in a life-limiting, rigid way that comes at a cost to your family.

Yet, the overall goal in Acceptance and Commitment Therapy (ACT)—and of this book—is to help people become more *psychologically flexible*, or be able to mindfully connect with the present moment and still pursue values-aligned behaviors and choices even when it's hard to do.[3] Being psychologically flexible means having the willingness to commit to staying on the surfboard (but flexible in how you do so) even when the waves try to throw you off. As an allergy parent, being psychologically flexible is having the willingness to experience all your thoughts and feelings, including the anxious and overwhelming ones, yet still choose to pursue uncomfortable values-aligned experiences that are safe enough in service of helping your child grow into a self-sufficient adult who can effectively manage their allergy. It's also important to note that part of being psychologically flexible is accepting that it is psychologically healthy to have both pleasant and unpleasant thoughts and feelings. In fact, experiencing both types of thoughts and feelings gives you a more full and enriched perspective on life.[4]

Pause and Practice: Consider All Possible Outcomes

Because anxious minds tend to rigidly focus on negative outcomes and worst-case-scenarios, it's important to remind your mind to be flexible and consider other possible outcomes for anxiety-inducing situations. For example, when you think of your child accidentally eating their allergen, your mind likely jumps to the conclusion that your child will experience anaphylaxis or even worse, become a fatality statistic. Maybe they will experience anaphylaxis, but maybe they won't—there are lots of factors that influence the severity of allergic reactions. Even so, your automatic perspective is likely a negative and catastrophizing one.

To help you practice perspective shifting so that it becomes a skill you can call on when you need it, use the accidental allergen ingestion scenario and consider the following three outcomes:

- the worst-case outcome
- the best-case outcome
- the most likely outcome.

The worst-case outcome is likely the one your mind thinks of first; it's what was previously mentioned—that your child experiences anaphylaxis or even worse, doesn't recover from it. The best-case and most ideal outcome might be that despite the accidental allergen ingestion, your child doesn't have an allergic reaction. Yet, the most likely outcome is that even if your child experiences anaphylaxis, their emergency action plan and self-administered epinephrine device will likely help the reaction resolve. (As you read this, your anxious mind might be saying, "But what if it doesn't, and my child dies?" Recognize that that's an anxious thought and remind yourself that thoughts are not outcome predictors. It may also feel helpful to revisit the fatality statistics presented in Chapter 2 and strategies for managing anxious thoughts described in Chapter 4.)

To help you practice perspective shifting so you can engage with more flexible perspectives rather than rigid ones, use this worst-case, best-case, and most likely

(*continued*)

outcome exercise anytime you notice yourself getting hooked by your anxious allergy-related thoughts or taking a tunnel-vision point of view. You can even practice it with other non-allergy situations that cause anxiety. Later in this chapter, I will share another strategy to help you practice perspective shifting when navigating overwhelming situations.

GAIN PERSPECTIVE ON WHO YOU ARE AS AN ALLERGY PARENT

Perspective shifting doesn't just mean developing different viewpoints about your experiences and the world around you; it also relates to your perspective on yourself. In fact, research shows that perspective shifting fosters the ability to unhook from negative thoughts and feelings about oneself, which makes it easier to practice self-compassion (rather than self-criticism)—a skill we will explore shortly.[5]

Cara reached out for therapy when she found herself struggling to follow the allergist's recommendation to introduce allergens to her infant daughter. Cara had kept the house peanut and egg-free since her three-year-old son had been diagnosed with peanut and egg allergies as an infant. Now that she was being encouraged to introduce peanut and egg (among other common allergens) to her infant daughter, she found herself terrified to do so. Cara wanted to follow the allergist's guidance, but thinking through the logistics of how to do so safely sent her into a tailspin. How could she have peanut and egg in her house and keep her son safe? What if her daughter could tolerate her son's allergens? How would she keep them in her daughter's diet while also keeping her son safe? The overwhelm was growing, and she wasn't making any progress toward meeting her allergen introduction goals since she just kept avoiding it. What's more, she realized that she had become self-critical about her inability to move forward with these introductions. She often noticed herself getting hooked by judgmental thoughts such as "Why can't you just follow the guidelines they've given you? Why are you being so ridiculous about this?"

At the onset of therapy, I helped Cara become clear about her allergy parenting goal: to introduce allergens to her daughter in a way that felt safe for her son and workable for her. Next, we discussed the developmentally focused allergy parenting goals for her daughter's current stage (which helped to reinforce why this was an important goal to pursue), identified unhelpful anxious thoughts and the mindset she was fused with (the "I Can't Do This" narrative), explored the allergy parenting trap she felt stuck in (the Over-Avoidance Trap), and identified the values she'd like to focus on in addition to safety (courage and persistence). Then I asked her to mindfully observe herself as an allergy parent and introduced her to the concept of *self-as-context* to help her do this.

In ACT, one of the hardest concepts to explain and understand is *self-as-context*. Also referred to as the *observing self* or *noticing self*, it means being able to view yourself through a lens that allows you to see all the parts of yourself, not just the unhelpful "I am" statements you've assigned to yourself (e.g., I am an ineffective allergy parent).[6] The goal with self-as-context is that you can mindfully and flexibly observe your internal content (thoughts and feelings), yet still have a stable, grounded, enduring sense of self that isn't defined by this content.[7] Being able to observe yourself also helps you to unhook from your inner critic (that voice that often tells you that you're not good enough) rather than staying stuck believing the unhelpful descriptions and judgmental thoughts that come to mind. To help my clients understand how to observe themselves more concretely, I share these two analogies: (1) It's as if you are watching yourself as a character on a television show, and (2) it's as though you can physically observe yourself by sitting in a chair and watching your internal thoughts and external actions at any given moment in time.

Being able to gain perspective on who you are as an allergy parent is just as important, if not more important than flexibly viewing your experiences. There are two key benefits of becoming an observer of yourself:

- It helps you become less attached to the *conceptualized self*, or the self-focused (and often critical) statements that you may use to describe yourself (e.g. I am not good at allergy parenting).[8] As previously mentioned, these concepts, which directly impact your choices and actions, form by letting your internal experiences (thoughts and feelings), labels (judgments), and narratives (the stories you tell yourself about yourself) define your identity. For instance, if you believe the "I'm not a good enough allergy parent, so I won't be able to keep my child safe" narrative that may be playing on repeat in your mind, then you're more likely to experience a lack of trust in your own allergy parenting choices and engage in unhelpful second-guessing and reassurance-seeking actions, which further fuels the sense of overwhelm.
- It also encourages you to engage in *self-compassion* rather than self-criticism when navigating challenging experiences. We'll explore this concept shortly, but

practicing self-compassion involves giving yourself the comfort, support, and understanding you'd offer a friend when you're struggling, suffering, and feeling bad about yourself.[9]

DEVELOPING A FLEXIBLE PERSPECTIVE ON WHO YOU ARE AS AN ALLERGY PARENT

Becoming an observer of yourself is a crucial skill to develop because your perspective on allergy parenting and how you feel about yourself as an allergy parent have a bidirectional relationship; that is, one influences the other. Therefore, having a stable sense of self that endures through challenging experiences makes it less likely that you'll take an inflexible, tunnel-vision view of yourself. This stable sense of self will also give you more confidence to pursue meaningful behavior changes that will allow you to adjust your perspective on allergy parenting from one that feels too overwhelming to one that feels possible to navigate.

When I asked Cara how she would describe herself as an allergy parent, she said that she noticed feeling sad. She had realized that the first description that came to mind wasn't kind ("I am an overwhelmed, anxious allergy parent who can't make decisions about how to effectively navigate stressful food allergy-related situations"). While struggling to introduce allergens to her infant daughter, her view of herself as an allergy parent, which was initially a favorable one, had changed to one that was based on her perceived shortcomings. Her self-talk was focused on self-blame, shame, and criticism ("Why can't you just follow the guidelines they've given you? Why are you being so ridiculous about this?"). It quickly became clear to me that she had developed tunnel vision—focusing only on this current challenge and basing her view of herself as an allergy parent on the unhelpful labels she had recently assigned herself. But I wanted her to widen her perspective by noticing and reconnecting with a variety of experiences thus far in her allergy parenting journey, not just this current experience. To do that, Cara and I worked through an exercise I call *watching your allergy parenting highlights reel*.

Pause and Practice: Watch Your Allergy Parenting Highlights Reel

If someone asked you to describe yourself as an allergy parent, what description would you give? What words and phrases would you use to describe the way in which you approach allergy parenting? Would you be judgmental and label yourself as an "anxious allergy parent" (as Cara did) simply because you experience anxious thoughts? Or would you use your values as the foundation for how you'd describe yourself as an allergy parent? For example, during an allergy-related challenge like the one that Cara was navigating, you might choose to describe yourself in the following compassionate and values-aligned way: "I'm a loving allergy parent who is still learning how to navigate difficult experiences."

To help you develop the ability to observe yourself rather than define yourself based on your internal "I am" statements, I want you to envision that you're watching a video on your computer or television. The video you're watching is a highlights reel of different experiences you've had so far in your allergy parenting journey. The video clips show a variety of different experiences—ones in which you felt overwhelmed and were unsure how to navigate, ones in which you felt you navigated things well, and ones in which you could see yourself growing as an allergy parent. Remember, the mind tends to recall negative and traumatic experiences more readily than it does seemingly less dramatic neutral or positive experiences, so it's important to actively reconnect with the neutral and positive images to help you consider multiple perspectives.

Envision yourself watching this video, as if you're watching a character in a show, and see what you notice about yourself in each clip. Specifically observe the following things:

- What rigid, rule-governed thoughts are you noticing (e.g., my child can't be safe outside of the home)?
- Are you using a tunnel-vision or panoramic perspective?
- Are you getting hooked by anxious thoughts about life with allergies?
- Can you notice what values are guiding your choices and actions?
- Are you engaging in values-aligned committed actions even when uncomfortable thoughts, feelings, or memories arise?
- What beliefs do you have about what it means to be a good allergy parent and keep your child safe?

(*continued*)

- Do these beliefs help or hinder your ability to take a relaxed readiness, values-aligned approach to life with allergies?

Next, consider what a consistent, yet flexible description of yourself as an allergy parent would be—one that is defined by focusing on multiple clips (and pieces of context) rather than on just one specific experience (which is likely a negative one). In other words, zoom out to widen your perspective. Finally, consider if this new description sits well with you. Does it align with the vision you had for yourself as a parent, and more specifically, an allergy parent? If not, why?

If you find that your description is still based on your unhelpful internal "I am" statements or that you're unable to take an observer stance, revisit and practice the cognitive defusion strategies in Chapter 4. These will help you to unhook from rigid thoughts so that you can shift perspectives and more clearly notice your values, which will help you form a more stable and enduring sense of self as an allergy parent.

TOOLS TO HELP YOU DEVELOP MORE FLEXIBLE PERSPECTIVES

Language

The language you use for both your internal self-talk and in conversations with others can influence your perspective and your mindset about parenting a child with allergies. In addition, the language you use can either help or hinder your ability to unhook from unhelpful anxious thoughts.

Have you ever paused to notice the tone of language and the phrases you use to discuss allergies, especially when you feel anxious? Do you speak about allergies using rigid, fear-based phrases, which includes words such as *should*, *must*, *always*, and *never*? Or are you able to use more flexible language, which includes words such as *might*, *could*, *maybe*, and *yet*?

For example, consider what tone and phrasing you'd use when thinking about making mistakes in allergy parenting (which happens because you're human), such as accidentally feeding your child a food that has their allergen as an ingredient or forgetting their inhaler. You might notice rigid, unhelpful language such as "I can't ever make mistakes," implying that mistakes in allergy parenting are always catastrophic (which isn't accurate). Or maybe you'd notice more flexible language that helps you shift your perspective, such as "If I make a mistake, I know how to handle it."

As you continue developing mindful awareness of your anxious thoughts, mindset, parenting traps, and values, pause to notice the overall tone of your language, as well as common words and phrases used when talking about allergies internally, with your child, and with others. Pay attention to how often you're using inflexible words such as *or* rather than the more flexible *and*; the former skews your perspective by creating an unhelpful "this or that" mentality. But don't worry if you notice yourself using rigid, fear-based language; you can learn to use more flexible language and then teach this skill to your child, too. To help you connect with and practice using more flexible language, consider the strategies in the "Pause and Practice" section.

Pause and Practice: Using Flexible Phrases to Help Shift Your Perspective

Think about an allergy-related scenario or situation that makes you feel overwhelmed or anxious. Maybe it's the thought of your child having an allergic reaction or asthma attack. Or perhaps it's an upcoming age and stage transition, such as starting at a new school. Use the flexible phrases below to help you unhook from these rigid thoughts and to shift to a more flexible perspective that allows you to consider multiple potential outcomes.

- **What if → If, then:** When noticing anxious *what-if* thoughts (e.g., What if my child has an allergic reaction?), flip that thought to be an *if, then* thought (e.g., If my child has an allergic reaction, then I will follow their emergency action plan and use their self-administered epinephrine device if necessary). Using *if, then* language helps turn *what-if* thoughts from unhelpful anxious thoughts into solution-focused plans of action.
- **What if → Even so:** Like shifting from *what-if* thoughts to *if, then* thoughts, flipping *what-if* thoughts to *even so* thoughts allows you to consider more flexible options and outcomes. For instance, you can turn "What if I feel anxious when bringing my child to a restaurant?" into "I may feel anxious when bringing my child to a restaurant, but even so, I can do it while feeling anxious if we've established that it's safe enough."

- **Can't → Yet:** When noticing rigid thoughts implying that you're incapable of something (e.g., I can't trust my own allergy parenting instincts), add the word *yet* to turn that thought into a more flexible one (e.g., I can't trust my own allergy parenting instincts yet). You can also add the word *yet* to turn a fixed mindset thought (I don't know how to evaluate allergy-related risks) into a growth mindset thought that implies you're still learning and developing skills (e.g., I don't know how to evaluate allergy-related risks yet).
- **Control → Influence:** When noticing control-focused thoughts (e.g., I need to control every possible risk if we eat out at a restaurant), reformulate that thought with a focus on influencing outcomes rather than aiming to control everything, which isn't possible to do (e.g., How can I influence things while eating out at a restaurant to help keep my child safe enough?). Similar to *if, then*, the word *influence* helps you brainstorm solution-focused actions rather than ruminate on the unhelpful (and impossible) goal of controlling everything around you.

Self-Compassion

As previously mentioned, Cara noticed that her self-talk was filled with judgmental language and that she had labeled herself as an overwhelmed, anxious allergy parent simply because she was struggling to begin allergen introductions. She no longer thought of herself as a capable allergy parent and now believed that feeling anxious and overwhelmed meant that she wasn't doing a good job with allergy parenting. Cara's perspective on herself as an allergy parent was clearly based on her unhelpful "I am" statements rather than on her values and the insights she gained from observing herself across various experiences.

Like Cara, you may find yourself being super critical of yourself as you reflect on what kind of allergy parent you are, so let's explore how self-compassion plays a role in learning how to be kinder to yourself, which helps you to live in alignment with your values and engage in more flexible perspectives.

Compassion's main purpose is to help alleviate suffering and to show care and concern for those who are struggling and experiencing emotional pain, which means that self-compassion is about caring for yourself when you're having these same experiences.[10] Practicing self-compassion helps you to use a growth mindset and build resiliency and can have positive impacts on your physical health and emotional well-being. The three main components of self-compassion are: *self-kindness*, *mindfulness*, and *common humanity*. *Self-kindness* means taking a warm and supportive approach to yourself to help put yourself in a better state of mind to cope with challenges. *Mindfulness* means being aware of and nonjudgmentally accepting all thoughts and feelings without ignoring or trying to control them. *Common humanity* helps you normalize your experiences by reminding yourself that you're not the only person wrestling with thoughts and feelings of inadequacy and imperfection, especially during challenging experiences.

Think of self-compassion as the antidote to self-criticism. In her book *Fierce Self-Compassion*, researcher Kristin Neff shares that when your self-concept is threatened, it's common to fight yourself with criticism and shame in hopes that you'll get rid of your perceived weakness by being forced to change.[11] The problem with pursuing behavior change by engaging in self-criticism is that even if you're temporarily motivated to make the change, being in a constant state of self-focused negativity can take a toll on your physical and mental health and emotional well-being. Therefore, being hard on yourself isn't the motivational strategy you'll want to use if you're pursuing meaningful changes in your allergy parenting approaches.

You may be wondering if self-compassion is the same thing as self-care. Even though as an allergy parent it's important to practice both, they're not the same thing, but they are related. *Self-compassion* is having an attitude of kindness and consideration for yourself, especially when experiencing pain and struggle, whereas *self-care* is engaging in kind and compassionate actions aimed at prioritizing your well-being. Practicing self-care might include engaging in good sleep and eating habits to ensure your optimal well-being and functioning, exercising and moving your body to help you effectively cope with tension and stress, and doing self-soothing activities aimed at inducing calmness and relaxation such as taking a warm bath. Examples of self-compassion practices include responding to yourself with supportive self-talk statements, doing mindfulness exercises to help formulate flexible perspectives, and pausing for deep breaths to offer yourself physical support.

One final note: Practicing self-compassion and self-care isn't selfish. On the contrary, when we're kinder to ourselves, we're often kinder to others. After all, you can't pour from an empty cup, so make sure your allergy parenting cup includes self-compassion and self-care.

Pause and Practice: Would I Say This to a Friend?

One of the easiest ways to assess whether you're practicing self-compassion during challenging experiences is to consider how you'd respond to yourself versus someone else in the same situation.

For example, if Cara was your friend and shared with you how difficult allergen introductions felt and that she was shaming herself for struggling with this process, how would you respond? What would you say? What tone would your message have—compassionate or critical? Would you offer her a hug? Would you jump to assumptions about Cara based on her struggle to introduce allergens? I'd guess that you'd take a compassionate approach, encouraging her to be kinder and more patient with herself rather than continuing to engage in self-judgment.

Now, imagine you were in that same situation. What would you say to yourself? What tone would your self-talk statements have—compassionate or critical? What assumptions would you make about yourself? Would you blame yourself for delaying allergen introductions, and if so, what "I am" statements would form from that self-blame?

Through this exercise, you likely noticed that you'd approach Cara differently than you'd approach yourself in the same situation. If so, you're not alone. Many don't hesitate to act compassionately toward others, yet they don't apply the same compassion to themselves when they're in similar situations. Instead, they engage in self-criticism, judgment, blame, and shame, which pushes people to stay hooked by unhelpful anxious thoughts and "I am" statements. It also skews your ability to gain perspective and leads to overestimating negative outcomes. None of this helps allergy parents manage the overwhelm.

If you find that you're compassionate toward others, but not as compassionate toward yourself, begin working toward changing this pattern by engaging in the following strategies, especially when you notice yourself being self-critical:

- **Turn self-critical "I am" statements into self-compassionate ones.** For instance, turn "I'm ridiculous for not being able to do these allergen introductions" into "I'm finding it hard to introduce these allergens—but I can be patient with myself as I would be for someone else."
- **Practice physical compassion.** Start by placing your hand on your heart to feel the warmth. Then take two or three deep belly breaths, engaging both your chest and belly as you inhale and exhale. As you're doing this, ask yourself what you need to do to show yourself compassionate support. Incorporating compassionate touch to this mindful breathing exercise is key since research shows that the body responds to physical touch almost immediately, releasing oxytocin (the love hormone) and endorphins (the feel-good hormones), which help you feel supported and induce a sense of calmness.[12] Other options for practicing physical compassion include hugging yourself and gently stroking your hand or arm.

GAINING PERSPECTIVE SO YOU CAN ACT MORE FLEXIBLY

Allergy parents often find themselves on a quest to find *the perfect* allergy management guidance that will make it nearly impossible to have allergic reactions or asthma attacks. Many parents I've worked with have said, "I just want someone to tell me *exactly* what to do (and not do) to keep my child safe!"

It makes sense that allergy parents tend to crave very clear rules and rigid guidelines—this makes them feel more in control and less anxious. But even if the perfect, fool-proof allergy management guidance *did* exist, does inflexibly following allergy management guidelines truly help allergy parents feel less overwhelmed? I would argue no. While rigidly following allergy management guidelines as perfectly as you'd follow directions on a map or steps in a recipe might lessen anxiety in the short term, it can open the door to challenges in the long term, including

- limiting your ability to develop competence and confidence in your own allergy parenting skills
- stunting the development of (and trust in) your own parenting instincts, leaving you to second-guess your actions and struggle with feelings of self-doubt
- limiting your willingness to adjust allergy management approaches as your child grows older, thereby impacting their developmental and social health
- limiting life experiences due to the unhelpful belief that allergy management guidelines require you to avoid all situations that aren't allergen-free

- creating a false sense of security, or the belief that perfectly following the guidelines means that there will never be an allergic reaction or asthma attack
- impacting your sense of self as an allergy parent when mistakes happen or when you can't perfectly follow allergy guidelines.

I'm not suggesting that allergy parents ignore allergy management guidance; on the contrary, you should follow the evidence-based allergy management guidelines given to you by your allergist. What I'm suggesting is that *how* you follow these guidelines is what matters. More specifically, I'm suggesting that you should aim to apply these guidelines in workable ways that allow for engaging in values-aligned living, meeting developmental goals, and practicing skills to create confidence in your (and your child's) ability to handle allergy-related emergencies. If you think of life with allergies as a puzzle, where pieces have only one spot where they fit perfectly, then you'll be focused on making *your life* fit into the allergy management guidelines rather than making *the guidelines* fit into your life.

What's more, adding allergy management guidelines into your life (rather than the other way around) encourages you to engage in more flexible (rather than rigid) actions that are determined by your values and parenting goals, not by the fear of making a misstep. Acting more flexibly may feel like you're giving up control, which can seem terrifying, but remember that you can't have complete control over anything, so that shouldn't be the goal. Remember also that you don't have to avoid everything that makes you anxious; you can keep your child safe while also engaging in life's experiences. So, keep in mind that it's more useful to focus on how you can influence situations and their outcomes through allergy education, skill-building, evaluating situations effectively, using problem-solving-focused language, and being willing to flexibly change your mind (and perspective) if something is no longer workable.[13]

Let's explore two common food allergy-related scenarios and how to navigate them with a flexible (rather than rigid) perspective so you can take flexible, values-aligned actions.

- **Conflict with schools about allergy management:** It can feel terrifying to send your child to school, especially if the administrators seem unwilling to cooperate on developing workable allergy management protocols. When this is the case, your anxious mind might want you to double down on your desired protocols without much conversation, but here's a more flexible, values-aligned way to navigate this scenario. First, have your allergist help you define what allergy management strategies are necessary for keeping your child safe, as these decisions are not one-size-fits all. As part of this discussion, identify which items are non-negotiable safety items and which items you might be more flexible with. (For instance, maybe having the whole class wash their hands after lunch isn't feasible, but using handwipes is an option.) Having this information from your allergist is important because when emotions (especially anxiety) are in the lead, it's more likely that you'll end up in a standoff with the school than making progress in a collaborative effort, which is the goal. So, focus on using evidence-based, solution-focused language, which helps with conflict resolution. Use open-ended, problem-solving questions such as

"What *can* be done?" when experiencing pushback. Remember, both allergy parents and school administrators want agency in the decision-making process, so being firm but kind goes a long way when trying to develop a workable, collaborative relationship. Stay connected with how you want to show up as an allergy parent and what your goal is—to keep your child safe yet allow them opportunities for developmental growth. Finally, if you and the school are unable to develop a workable plan, talk with your allergist about how best to proceed, including exploring alternate options.

- **Eating out and traveling:** Remember, an anxious mind will push you to avoid situations that make you feel uncomfortable, convincing you that they're unsafe even if they're not. To help you consider different perspectives on feared experiences such as eating out and traveling so that you can engage in flexible, values-aligned actions, start by talking with your allergist to gain clarity on your child's allergy-related risks and how to navigate these scenarios safely. Next, using that insight as your foundation, consider flexible actions that will allow you to safely engage in important experiences, such as traveling to see friends and family and eating meals outside of the home. For instance, to safely eat outside of the home, seek out allergy-friendly restaurants and develop a safety checklist and a conversation script to help you assess safety with the restaurant manager. These days it's easy to find menus online, too, so you can check in advance to help you prepare ahead of time. You might also decide to bring food from home so your child can eat safely if restaurants aren't allergy friendly. For traveling, consider bringing your own food, especially for airline travel, and look for vacation rentals or hotels that have kitchens. Considering and pursuing flexible actions encourage you to take a different perspective on experiences you may have previously avoided out of fear rather than necessity.

As I wrap up this chapter, I want to return to Cara. The allergen introduction experience was an opportunity for her not only to gain a more flexible perspective on herself as an allergy parent, but also to practice taking flexible perspectives and then acting more flexibly. Throughout this whole process, Cara often had to remind herself to stay connected with her multiple values, to focus on influencing outcomes rather than seeking control, and to remember why she was committed to introducing allergens to her daughter.

After clarifying her allergy parenting goal, I helped Cara work toward accepting that introducing allergens may feel uncomfortable, but were purposeful, values-aligned actions to pursue. Next, Cara practiced shifting perspectives by reminding herself that discomfort doesn't automatically mean something is unsafe, which helped her to consider more flexible outcomes, not just the ones she feared. Then we worked on noticing other unhelpful anxious thoughts that were pushing her to avoid introducing allergens so she could respond to those differently as well. Once Cara started practicing self-compassion by changing the tone of her internal self-talk and engaging in more self-care activities, she was better able to unhook from the self-judgmental "I am" statements by responding with compassionate, empowering, and values-aligned self-talk. (*Of course, this feels hard, as it does for other parents. But I can be brave and do hard things for the benefit of my child.*) All of this allowed her to develop a more stable sense of self that was based on her observations and values rather than on her perceived shortcomings.

A few years after we ended therapy, Cara reached back out with an update. While anxiety and overwhelm continued to be present during challenging experiences, Cara shared that learning the skills we covered in therapy had helped her to become a more mindful allergy parent and helped her learn how to regain a balanced perspective when challenges arose. What's more, Cara shared that learning how to practice self-compassion made such an empowering impact on her life that it's a skill she consistently encourages other allergy parents to practice, too, especially those whose children are newly diagnosed.

TAKEAWAYS

- Developing alternative perspectives helps you become more psychologically flexible, unhook from unhelpful anxious thoughts, and take values-aligned flexible actions even in the face of allergy parenting challenges.
- It's helpful to practice developing perspectives on yourself as an allergy parent, as well as your allergy parenting experiences and challenges.
- Self-compassion is the antidote to self-criticism. Practicing self-compassion helps you engage in a growth mindset and build resiliency during the allergy parenting journey.

Think About and Do

- How will you remind yourself to shift perspectives when you're seeing things through a tunnel-vision perspective?
- What will help you remember to consider multiple possible outcomes for challenging and anxiety-inducing situations (e.g., worst-case, best-case, most likely outcomes)? Are there any specific allergy-related situations to which you can apply this practice currently?
- Consider how practicing self-compassion will impact how you feel about allergy parenting. Will it help you feel less pressure to be a perfect allergy parent, and help you unhook from the unhelpful thought that you can't make mistakes?
- Choose one or two self-compassion statements that you're willing to practice consistently using and especially when allergy parenting feels hard or when mistakes are made.

CHAPTER 7

Putting Your Balanced, Mindful Allergy Parenting Plan into Action

At the beginning of this book, I asked you to answer this question: *Would I parent differently if my anxiety and fear didn't have a hold on me or push me around?*

Given that you are reading this book, I'm guessing you answered "yes" to that question. And I hope that by now, you're feeling a sense of relief that there are strategies to help you parent the way you want to rather than the way your anxious mind tells you to. I also hope that you not only see how parenting mindfully will help you navigate the overwhelm and unhook from anxiety, but that you feel ready to put these strategies into action and find a more balanced approach to parenting a child with allergies.

To help you do this, let's quickly review what was covered, look at stories of two parents who transitioned from parenting anxiously to parenting mindfully, and then work through exploratory questions that will make it easier for you to develop your mindful allergy parenting plan so that you can begin to put it into practice today.

COMMON FACTORS THAT CONTRIBUTE TO THE OVERWHELM IN ALLERGY PARENTING

The obvious answer to the question "What makes parents of children managing allergies feel overwhelmed?" are the diagnoses and the challenges that accompany living with them. But as you've learned from reading this book, beyond the diagnosis itself, many factors lead parents of children with allergies to feeling overwhelmed.

When parenting a child with allergies, it's easy to become *psychologically inflexible*, or to let your anxiety push you into a struggle with uncomfortable thoughts and feelings, and then engage in control-seeking behaviors as a way of dealing with them. When this happens, you're also more likely to overestimate allergy-related risks and interpret everything as unsafe for your child and thus will likely respond by avoiding life experiences beyond what's necessary to keep your child safe. All this fuels the overwhelm rather than defuses it.

What helps allergy parents navigate the overwhelm is by becoming more *psychologically flexible*, which begins with acknowledging all thoughts and feelings and purposefully choosing actions that are rooted in your values and allergy parenting goals rather than repeating what's not working well. Becoming more *psychologically flexible* not only helps you adapt to life's many changes; it's also a key component of mental health and well-being, helping to decrease stress and anxiety and improve confidence. Even though it may feel hard at first to practice being more psychologically flexible, it's worth the benefits it provides.

Just as your emotional well-being benefits from living in a *psychologically flexible* way, so does taking a *relaxed readiness approach* to allergy management. Taking a *relaxed readiness approach* doesn't mean that you'll be hands-off and miss important safety warnings, thereby leading to more allergic reactions or asthma attacks (although, your anxious mind might try to convince you of this). On the contrary, and as we covered in Chapter 3, taking a *relaxed readiness approach* means finding a workable balance between living in fear and living fully. It allows you to learn how to engage in a "just right" amount of caution (rather than an excessive amount that fuels debilitating anxiety), all while being prepared to address allergic reactions as you, your child, and your family engage in life's experiences rather than excessively avoiding them out of fear.

Here's a quick review of common factors that contribute to the overwhelm in allergy parenting to help reinforce which ones might be impacting you before you begin working on developing your mindful allergy parenting plan.

Anxiety and fear. Anxiety is a normal human emotion that everyone experiences, but also one that often makes us feel uncomfortable—physically and emotionally. Because anxiety encourages you to look ahead and worry about future-focused situations, it makes it hard to stay focused on the here and now, which further fuels anxiety. When fearful of something that could imminently endanger your child's health, safety, and well-being, such as an allergic reaction or asthma attack, your body will likely respond to this stress by going into *fight or flight* mode so that you're ready to act swiftly. This can happen even when you're just thinking about a threat to their safety or when you perceive something to be a threat even if it's not. Additionally, sometimes parents can stay in *fight or flight* or high alert mode indefinitely when they're constantly ruminating on their allergy worries, making it harder to accurately assess allergy-related risks. As we covered in Chapter 4, when dealing with perceived (not actual) threats, which likely happens often, it's important to help your mind unhook (cognitively defuse) from these fear-based thoughts and to help your body return to *rest and digest* mode so it can calm down and you can think clearly again.

Navigating uncertainty and unpredictability: Speaking of anxious minds and fear, the sense of unpredictability and uncertainty associated with allergic conditions often leaves allergy parents feeling very anxious and anticipating worst-case outcomes, especially when it comes to allergic reactions and asthma attacks. To induce a sense of calm, anxious minds like to know exactly what to do and what to expect, as well as reassurance that everything will be okay. As we covered in Chapter 2, where we explored parenting traps, it makes sense that allergy parents are often in the pursuit of certainty to calm their anxiety. Unfortunately, part of adjusting to life with allergies (and life in general) is accepting the uncertainties and the fact that you won't have control over everything. Instead, you'll want to focus on positively influencing outcomes by being informed, practicing allergy management skills, and preparing for a variety of situations and outcomes.

Lack of information and clarity: Two of the biggest sources of uncertainty are (1) lack of information and (2) lack of clarity. When you don't have enough information (especially on daily management, assessing allergy-related risks, and allergy safety strategies) or you don't have a clear, workable plan for how to keep your child safe, your mind is going to push you to find that clarity anywhere you can—usually online, which can fuel anxiety instead. What's more, since there's no one right way to manage allergies, as many factors impact how families manage these diagnoses, it's important that the information and clarity you're seeking are specific to your child's allergy and your family dynamics. Thus, the foundation for dealing with the overwhelm and anxiety associated with allergy parenting is working with a board-certified allergist who uses current best practices for patient care and whom you trust, as well as engaging with evidence-based, reputable information sources. As we covered in Chapter 2, the source of online allergy information matters, as does understanding how various types of information can help or hinder your ability to manage allergy parenting overwhelm. The core of your allergy information should come from your allergist and from online sources sharing *evidence-based information*, which is derived from available research and shared by qualified professionals. *Lived experience–based information*, which consists of personal experiences and is often what's shared in online allergy groups, can help you gain different perspectives on allergy parenting, but your allergy management and parenting decisions shouldn't be based on this type of information as every family's allergy profile and application of management approaches are unique.

Previous allergic reactions and asthma attacks: Whether it was your experience of your child's diagnosis (as was the case with my son) or of subsequent allergic reactions or asthma attacks, these experiences often feel like a setback for parents because they're traumatic and stir the uncertainty pot again. As we covered in Chapter 1, parents experience (and often struggle with) many emotions after diagnosis and subsequent reactions, which lead to the development of internal narratives that can increase the overwhelm for parents of children with allergies. It's not uncommon for anxiety and overwhelm to increase after your child has a reaction, but that doesn't mean you can't or won't work your way back to parenting mindfully and taking a *relaxed readiness approach* to allergy management again. Give yourself time and heavy doses of self-compassion as you work through the strategies in this book, which are not only helpful in establishing your mindful allergy parenting path, but also in reestablishing it after setbacks. Remember, setbacks are inevitable, so don't interpret them as a sign that you've done something wrong or that you're not a good enough allergy parent. Also, if you find yourself struggling to move forward after your child has an allergic reaction or asthma attack, I've shared tips and resources for finding licensed mental health practitioners in the resource section at the end of this book.

Navigating age and stage transitions: Adjusting to parenting a child with allergies takes time, information-gathering, developing (and practicing) allergy management skills, and accepting that you will inevitably need to readjust multiple times when life throws new factors into the mix (and it will). It's understandable to feel frustrated when you've finally gained confidence in your allergy parenting capabilities and something new, such as your child entering school or having new experiences, shakes that confidence. In Chapter 3, we explored key developmental stages and allergy parenting goals to help you parent more mindfully and navigate the inevitable ups and downs as you work toward raising a self-sufficient adult who is increasingly able to manage their allergy on their own. It's also important to be aware of three developmental processes happening simultaneously: your child's development, your parental development, and the development of your allergy management approaches. When parenting anxiously, it's easy to lose sight of the need to delicately balance these three processes and to establish parenting goals, which helps you navigate the overwhelm and take a relaxed readiness approach to allergy management. As such, it's crucial to stay mindful of the bigger perspective (encouraging your child's growth and development throughout the years) while staying focused on their current age and stage so you don't hinder their skill-building and increase your overwhelm with debilitating anticipatory anxiety about future stages.

Fusion with unhelpful thoughts and beliefs: A major aspect of the overwhelm that many allergy parents experience is when unhelpful thoughts and beliefs lead decision-making, cloud perspective, and determine parenting and allergy management actions. As we covered in Chapter 4, *cognitive fusion* is when you've become so tightly intertwined with your thoughts that you can't separate yourself from or give yourself the ability to mindfully consider them and how you want to respond to them. Becoming hooked by your unhelpful anxious thoughts hinders your ability to be psychologically flexible. When this happens, it's as if you have tunnel vision and are unable to focus on any other thoughts (other than the ones you're fused with), notice what's happening in the world around you, and envision a workable path forward. It's no surprise that staying cognitively fused with anxious thoughts further fuels the overwhelm. In this case, the goal is to mindfully observe these thoughts and respond to them in ways that allow you to move in whatever direction you need to—hopefully a direction that allows you to balance the anxiety and a good quality of life.

Control-seeking goals and behaviors: Being hooked by anxious thoughts and unhelpful beliefs about life with allergies can lead allergy parents to engage in control-seeking goals and behaviors. The goals of these actions? To feel less anxious and create a sense of certainty where there might not otherwise be. Yes, you want to take actions aimed at keeping your child safe, but trying to control everything around you isn't a workable safety strategy long term, as it's impossible to have complete control. It also doesn't help with anxiety management in the long term because you'll feel more anxious and overwhelmed every time you can't control something, and ultimately may end up over-avoiding life's experiences. Instead, you can help decrease the overwhelm by thinking about how you can positively influence situations so that your child stays safe while also engaging in life's experiences.

Lack of connection with values: When feeling anxious and engaging in control-seeking behaviors, it's easy to experience a loss of connection with *values*, or the chosen actions and ways of living that are guided by what you find meaningful and important. More specifically, when focusing only on the value of safety (especially the all-or-nothing definition of safety), it's easy to ignore or overlook other important values and to restrict your child's opportunities to practice age-appropriate skills due to fear about their safety (which can negatively impact their social and emotional development). When disconnected from other important non-safety values, it's also easier for your anxious thoughts to push you back into parenting anxiously anytime you're facing a challenging situation. On the contrary, learning how to hold multiple values (rather than only focusing on safety) helps you navigate the overwhelm, as together, these values serve as a guide for how you want to parent your child. What's more, pairing values with developmentally focused parenting goals gives you a solid plan for parenting your child mindfully rather than anxiously. Finally, psychological flexibility and a relaxed readiness approach to allergy management are tools that help you engage in purposeful behaviors aimed at not only keeping your child safe, but also raising them to embody the characteristics that will allow them to bravely and confidently navigate the world with allergies.

USING MINDFUL ALLERGY PARENTING PRACTICES TO NAVIGATE THE OVERWHELM

Before you begin putting together your mindful allergy parenting plan, let's look at two parents who felt overwhelmed by many of the factors we just explored and how they used the strategies shared in this book to turn off anxiety autopilot and begin parenting more mindfully.

Naomi

Naomi's son Hunter, who has a peanut allergy and asthma, had attended a peanut-free preschool. Because it was a small, allergy-friendly school, all the staff were aware of Hunter's peanut allergy and asthma diagnoses and were trained in emergency protocols for both, which felt reassuring to Naomi. What's more, Hunter never felt excluded from birthday celebrations, and other parents often turned to Naomi to ask for peanut-free brand recommendations. Allergy parenting felt manageable during the preschool years.

However, weeks before Hunter was to begin kindergarten at a bigger school that wasn't peanut-free, she noticed her anxiety level increasing. While she and school administrators had developed a health plan with agreed-upon safety protocols, Naomi's mind kept focusing on worst case scenarios. *Because it's such a big school, what if not all the staff know who he is? What if he sits next to someone eating a PB&J sandwich and has an allergic reaction? What if he keeps getting sick and having asthma attacks because he's exposed to so many more kids? Maybe I should find a smaller school or homeschool him to keep him safe?* These kinds of anxious thoughts were on repeat around the clock; they even made her feel physically ill. In response to these thoughts, Naomi found herself staying up all night researching other school options because she had convinced herself that Hunter couldn't stay safe at such a big school. She also kept him home from the kindergarten meet up at the local park because she began to feel as though there were allergy-related risks and asthma triggers everywhere. On the suggestion of a fellow allergy parent, Naomi reached out for therapy to help her navigate the overwhelm that had started impacting her daily functioning and parenting.

First, we talked about how anxiety is a future-focused emotion that can cause parents to become hooked by their worries and unhelpful beliefs (e.g., my son won't be safe at a bigger school that isn't peanut-free). In addition, we discussed how anxiety can be useful if you employ mindful management strategies that help you develop a different relationship with it, strategies Naomi would learn in our work together. We also discussed how it's not uncommon for anxiety to increase during age and stage transitions (such as going to a new school) and how her control-seeking actions, such as avoiding the kindergarten playdate, may have temporarily lessened her anxiety, but would exacerbate it in the long-term.

Next, we discussed Naomi's understanding of her son's allergies, as worrying about accidental exposures was a substantial source of her overwhelm. It quickly became clear that many of Naomi's anxious thoughts stemmed from a lack of clarity about allergy-related risks. Because of this lack of clarity, Naomi started feeling more uncertain about Hunter's safety, interpreting everything as unpredictable and risky. What's more, even though Hunter's allergic reaction happened after ingesting peanuts, she had convinced herself that he would react just sitting next to someone eating his allergen even though this had never happened before. Under the circumstances, I encouraged Naomi to consult with her son's allergist to gain more information and clarity on allergy-related risks and safety to help her unhook from her anxious thoughts and to learn how to more effectively evaluate perceived versus actual risks specific to Hunter's allergy.

Using the information their allergist provided as the foundation, we began mapping out her mindful allergy parenting plan. First, Naomi identified that she was stuck in both the Certainty and Over-Avoidance Traps, which helped her to understand that the control-seeking behaviors she was engaging in that were aimed at decreasing her anxiety ultimately made it worse. Next, she changed her internal narrative from "My son won't be safe at school" to "The school and I have developed strategies to keep my son safe, including a plan for how to address any potential emergencies." Then I helped Naomi identify and focus on her current allergy parenting goals, which included nurturing Hunter's social and emotional health and guiding him as he developed more allergy management skills of his own. Reconnecting with these developmentally focused parenting goals helped Naomi shift her perspective from one focused solely on the value of safety to one that allowed her to prioritize multiple values, specifically connection (to grow friendships), courage (to engage in experiences rather than avoid them), and safety (to stay safe while having fun at school). When her anxious thoughts popped up, she would unhook from them by reminding herself they were just thoughts (and not outcome predictors), take deep calming breaths, and then thank her mind for trying to be helpful by saying, "Thank you for trying to make sure my son stays safe; we've got a good plan in place."

Of course, anxiety was still present while doing this work, so I reminded Naomi of another important perspective shift—that the goal wasn't to eliminate anxiety since there's no delete button for anxious thoughts; rather, the goal was to interact with anxiety in more workable ways so she could let her values and parenting goals lead the way forward. Yes, she still worried about Hunter's safety, but armed with these new tools, she related differently to her overwhelm about the upcoming transition and was better able to navigate her anxious thoughts. The morning Hunter started kindergarten, he told her how excited he was to meet his new classmates, and because she had been practicing her mindful parenting strategies, Naomi was able to be present (rather than hooked by her anxious thoughts) and felt excited for him, too. She also felt more empowered about navigating the overwhelm of future age and stage transitions now that she had a toolkit of mindful strategies to use.

John

John's son Mateo managed dairy and cashew allergies. A senior in high school, he was having the time of his life. Mateo went out with his friends most nights, but unfortunately, was inconsistent about carrying his self-administered epinephrine devices, often leaving the house without them. Of course, the lack of follow-through made John and his wife upset because they were afraid of what would happen if Mateo had an allergic reaction without his self-administered epinephrine devices. Both being pediatricians, John and his wife inundated themselves with food allergy–related research. Therefore, they knew that teens were more likely to engage in risky behaviors and considered not carrying self-administered epinephrine devices as one of those risky behaviors. Their fear led them to lecturing Mateo most nights and threatening to ground him in hopes of getting him to be more committed to carrying his self-administered epinephrine devices. But with each lecture, Mateo tuned his parents out and pulled farther away from them. What's more, not having had an allergic reaction since elementary school, he wasn't worried he'd have another one because he had managed to stay safe all these years. Therefore, Mateo felt his parents were being dramatic by constantly lecturing him about allergy safety.

After months of conflict and negative impacts on their parent-child relationships, the three of them began family therapy. Without realizing it, John and his wife had been stuck in the Over-Functioning Trap as a way of ensuring Mateo's safety. In response to the anxiety they felt after inundating themselves with food allergy–related research, they had been engaging in control-seeking actions including asking safety questions while out at restaurants (rather than Mateo self-advocating), taking control of medical appointments (rather than teaching Mateo how to navigate appointments and gaining agency), and carrying the self-administered epinephrine devices when out of the home (because they didn't trust him to remember them). This meant that Mateo hadn't been developing and practicing his allergy management skills.

We continued exploring and identifying the sources of their overwhelm, which included getting hooked by anxious thoughts, which pushed them to lose connection with other important values such as encouraging Mateo's responsibility and independence; their uncertainty about Mateo's ability to manage his allergies; responding to this uncertainty by overfunctioning, which fueled the overwhelm; and losing sight of two key parenting goals—helping Mateo become a self-sufficient young adult capable of managing his allergies well and keeping their parent-child relationships intact while doing so. With all these new insights, John and his wife gained a new perspective. They now understood how their control-seeking actions had impeded Mateo's ability to develop his own allergy management skills and that the lack of opportunities to practice self-management impacted Mateo's willingness to be responsible for his own allergy safety. On the flip side, Mateo also had a perspective shift, enabling him to understand that showing his parents he could be trusted by consistently carrying his self-administered epinephrine devices would result in a decrease in his parents' anxiety and less conflict between them.

Turning to more mindful approaches for navigating this conflict, John and his wife began practicing how to unhook from their own anxious thoughts by pausing and mindfully observing them. Next, they practiced purposefully responding to these thoughts with values-aligned actions that focused on encouraging Mateo's safety, as well as his independence and responsibility. One of these values-aligned actions included engaging in shared decision-making rather than lecturing, especially since Mateo said he would be more receptive to his parents' messages if they would engage in calm, two-way discussions in which he had the chance to be heard, too. Consequently, we practiced active listening techniques and sharing messages in a calm manner. We also discussed other values-aligned actions that would allow Mateo to develop his allergy management skills and show he could be trusted to do so with safety parameters set by his parents. Together, they established that Mateo would be responsible for developing a strategy that helped him to consistently remember his self-administered epinephrine devices, such as setting a reminder on his phone, and when he failed to remember them, he would have to stop whatever he was doing and come home to get them no matter how inconvenient it was.

Months after finishing therapy, John reached out with an update. He and his wife continued using their new mindful allergy parenting plan, which helped them unhook from anxious thoughts and regain perspective so they could pursue values-aligned actions rather than fear-based reactions. Their more mindful approaches and the use of the shared decision-making and communication strategies we discussed in therapy had led to a more connected relationship with Mateo. What's more, Mateo was now not only consistently carrying his self-administered epinephrine devices, but he was also asking for more opportunities to practice his allergy management skills and show his parents he could be trusted. While they weren't always aligned, John and his wife were committed to letting Mateo have input on allergy management strategies and opportunities to develop his management skills as long as he exhibited his trustworthiness by continuing to show effort and keeping the lines of communication open.

IT'S TIME TO CREATE YOUR MINDFUL ALLERGY PARENTING PLAN

Now that we've reviewed common factors that contribute to the overwhelm in allergy parenting, reiterated the overall goal of becoming more *psychologically flexible* and developing a *relaxed readiness approach* to allergy management, and explored how two parents made the switch to parenting more mindfully, it's time to help you create your own mindful allergy parenting plan.

In your journal, consider the topics described below to help you explore your current parenting approach and consider what a more mindful approach would look like. You can also list actionable ways in which you can work toward making these adjustments. Be as specific as possible with your answers, as they will serve as the foundation for your new mindful approach to allergy parenting. You can revisit this section and answer these questions anytime you feel anxiety autopilot turning back on to help you recommit to your mindful allergy parenting approach again.

Explore Your Allergy Parenting Narratives

As discussed in Chapter 1, identifying unhelpful beliefs and narratives impacting your perspective, as well as acknowledging whether you're engaging in a fixed mindset (e.g., I'm not capable of keeping my child safe) or a growth mindset (e.g., I can learn strategies for keeping my child safe) helps you work toward adjusting or formulating new, more empowering narratives.

Current approach:

- What unhelpful beliefs and narratives did you develop about allergy parenting after your child was diagnosed? Are these narratives still impacting how you parent today?
- List any other unhelpful narratives impacting how you currently parent.
- Are you subscribing to a fixed or growth mindset about allergy parenting?

Mindful approach:

- Write out new allergy parenting narratives that are growth-mindset and empowering—ones that will help you persevere through challenging moments in allergy parenting.
- How will you recognize if you lose connection with these new narratives or become hooked by unhelpful narratives again? What specific thoughts, feelings, actions, and outcomes will you notice?

Identify Your Allergy Parenting Traps

As we explored in Chapter 2, you may have unknowingly become stuck in allergy parenting traps, or behavioral patterns that seem helpful in the short term but create more struggle in the long term. Therefore, recognizing these patterns helps you choose to engage in more mindful actions based on your values and parenting goals rather than fear and anxiety.

Current approach:

- List any allergy parenting traps you're stuck in from Chapter 2, noting how they felt helpful in the short term, but aren't helping the overwhelm and anxiety in the long term.

- How has being stuck in these allergy parenting traps impacted yourself, your child, your family, and your relationships?

Mindful approach:

- How will you know if you become stuck in allergy parenting traps again in the future? What specific thoughts, feelings, actions, and outcomes will you notice?
- What self-talk statements can you engage with to empower yourself to stay out of these traps and choose mindful, values-aligned actions instead (which may initially feel harder to do)?

Evaluate Your Ability to Assess Allergy-Related Risks

As discussed throughout the book, having a solid understanding of your child's allergies and knowing how to assess actual versus perceived allergy-related risks are foundational for navigating allergy parenting overwhelm, as these help you determine when it's safe enough to step outside of your comfort zone in service of pursuing values-aligned experiences for yourself and your child.

Current approach:

- How do you currently determine what experiences are safe enough for your child?
- Do you find that you tend to assume most experiences are unsafe for your child?

- Do you currently feel that you know how to accurately assess allergy-related risks, or determine which are perceived and which are actual safety risks?

Mindful approach:

- What questions about assessing allergy-related risks would feel helpful to ask your child's allergist, including determining the difference between perceived and actual safety risks and deciding what experiences are safe enough?
- After gathering this information from your allergist, how will you help yourself commit to pursuing values-aligned experiences that feel outside of your comfort zone, but are deemed safe enough by your allergist? What self-talk statements will you use and which reminders of why you're pursuing these changes will you stay connected with?

Identify Developmentally Focused Allergy Parenting Goals

As explored in Chapter 3, being mindful of your allergy parenting goals and key tasks for each age and stage helps you work toward a relaxed readiness approach to allergy management and find a workable balance between three developmental processes happening simultaneously (child development, parental development, and allergy skill development).

Current approach:

- Are you currently mindful of the three developmental processes while parenting?
- What allergy parenting goals and tasks are you currently focused on for your child's age and stage?

- List the ways in which you're feeling misaligned with or are overlooking key allergy parenting goals for your child's current stage.

Mindful approach:

- What thoughts and reminders will help you remember to stay focused on the present moment (e.g., not thinking too far in the future)?
- Write down which allergy parenting goals and tasks you'd like to focus on for your child's current age and stage.
- What allergy management skills would you like to master and teach your child (or help them master) now and in the next stage, if you're entering that stage soon?
- What thoughts and reminders will help you remember to stay mindful of the need to nurture all three developmental processes during each stage?

Determine How You'll Respond to Anxious Thoughts

As discussed in Chapter 4, you likely try to control your anxious allergy-related thoughts by ignoring or avoiding them and therefore will benefit from using cognitive defusion strategies that will help you unhook from anxious thoughts. Unhooking from these thoughts allows you space to choose purposeful actions that are in service of your child's safety and growth rather than engaging with actions aimed at managing your anxiety and feelings of overwhelm.

Current approach:

- Write down common anxious allergy-related thoughts you ruminate (or worry) over.

- List the ways in which you've been responding to or experientially avoiding your anxious thoughts, including trying to control, ignore, or escape them.
- What experiential and emotional costs do you experience when you try to control, ignore, or escape your anxious thoughts (e.g., feeling exhausted, not living in and enjoying the present moment, not learning skills that help you manage anxiety, avoiding experiences)?

Mindful approach:

- How will you remind yourself to mindfully observe your anxious and uncomfortable allergy-related thoughts so that you can choose how to respond to them rather than let them push you around?
- What cognitive defusion strategies will you practice to help you unhook from your anxious allergy-related thoughts (e.g., apply mental appreciation, regard thoughts as thoughts rather than outcome predictors, say your thoughts out loud)?
- What specific strategies will you use to calm your anxious mind and body when you're feeling overwhelmed (e.g., observing anxious thoughts, box breathing, physical movement)?

Connect or Reconnect with Multiple Values

As explored in Chapter 5, you may find yourself focusing only on the value of safety, especially all-or-nothing safety when parenting a child with allergies, and therefore will benefit from identifying or reconnecting with multiple values (or meaningful ways of living) to help guide you, your child, and your family through challenging experiences with a balance between living safely and living fully.

Current approach:

- List your current allergy parenting values—are there other values leading your parenting choices besides safety?
- List important-to-you values you've forgotten to consider or stay connected with in your current allergy parenting approach.

Mindful approach:

- List all your allergy parenting values and family values to use as guides as you engage in a more mindful allergy parenting approach (see your lists from Chapter 5).
- What will remind you to engage in an ***and*** mindset (so you can act in service of multiple values) rather than an ***or*** mindset (only focusing on one value)?
- Begin prioritizing which values will help you to pursue developmentally focused parenting goals and navigate challenging experiences. (Remember, you can adjust your list of prioritized values whenever needed.)

Engage in Values-Aligned Committed Action

As also discussed in Chapter 5, engaging in values-aligned committed action will help you act in service of your child's health and safety while also being mindful of important developmentally focused allergy parenting goals and effectively balancing all three important developmental processes.

Current approach:

- What actions do you currently engage in that align only with safety, especially all-or-nothing safety, or don't allow you to align with multiple values?

Mindful approach:

- How can you engage in committed action in service of multiple values at the same time?
- How will you know if you're focusing only on safety and ignoring your other values?
- Think of one or two specific scenarios in which you'd like to start acting in service of your child's safety and another important value (such as bravery, connection, independence, resilience, or responsibility). How will you begin working toward these goals?
- What are your whys, or reminders of why committed action is worthwhile even when it feels hard to pursue?

Practice Perspective Shifting

As explored in Chapter 6, gaining an understanding of your perspective on allergy parenting as a whole and of yourself as an allergy parent and then learning how to shift these perspectives helps you become more psychologically flexible so that you can effectively navigate the ups and downs of allergy parenting.

Current approach:

- Revisit your current perspectives on yourself and allergy parenting. Are these perspectives guided by tunnel vision (which is rigid) or panoramic views (which are broader and more inclusive)?

- What "I am" statements are you using to define yourself as an allergy parent? What pieces of context are you forgetting to consider as you take a broader view of yourself (e.g. your loving nature, your growth as an allergy parent, your willingness to step outside of your comfort zone)?
- Are you able to consider flexible outcomes in challenging situations and experiences (e.g., worst-case outcome, best-case outcome, most likely outcome), and if not, why?

Mindful approach:

- List more flexible, self-compassionate perspectives on yourself and allergy parenting.
- What flexible actions would you like to engage in, and how will these new perspectives help you to do so?
- How will you remind yourself to consider multiple outcomes when feeling anxious?
- How will you remind yourself to practice flexible self-talk phrases to help you shift perspectives when you're hooked by your anxious thoughts (e.g., turning *what-if* thoughts into *if, then* or *even so* thoughts and focusing on influence rather than control)?
- How will you engage in self-compassion and self-care? What actions will you take and what kinder self-talk statements will you use?

FINAL THOUGHTS

While some parents adjust to their child's diagnosis with ease, many others find the adjustment difficult for the very reasons covered in this book—even I did. Therefore, no matter how overwhelmed you feel on this allergy parenting journey, remember that you're not alone. Many other parents are experiencing the same thoughts and feelings as you.

I want to applaud your willingness to read this book and commit to making changes so that parenting a child with allergies feels less overwhelming and life feels more joy-filled for you, your child, and your family. It's an honor that you chose this book to help you navigate these emotional waves. I hope the insights, strategies, and tools shared in it will help you develop a more balanced perspective and mindful approach to allergy parenting. Remember, you can revisit and review the insights in this book as often as needed along the way.

If you've found this book helpful and want more evidence-based tips from me, including printables relating to this book, visit the Food Allergy Counselor website at www.FoodAllergyCounselor.com, where you'll find my articles, worksheets, podcast, and other resources. There, you can also learn how to work with me and how to sign up for my emails, which share practical insights and information about webinars and workshops.

Finally, I love connecting with families managing allergies, so please don't hesitate to reach out through my website to let me know how this book impacted you. It would be an honor to hear from you!

NOTES

Introduction

1. American Academy of Allergy, Asthma & Immunology (AAAI), "Allergies Symptoms, Diagnosis, Management & Treatment," n.d, accessed October 3, 2023, https://www.aaaai.org/conditions-treatments/allergies/allergies-overview.
2. Hyeong Yun Kim, Eun Byul Kwon, Ji Hyeon Baek, et al., "Prevalence and Comorbidity of Allergic Diseases in Preschool Children," *Korean Journal of Pediatrics* 56, no. 8 (2013): 338. https://doi.org/10.3345/kjp.2013.56.8.338.
3. R. S. Gupta, C. M. Warren, B. M. Smith, et al., "The Public Health Impact of Parent-Reported Childhood Food Allergies in the United States," *Pediatrics* 143, no. 3 (March 1, 2019),142(6):E20181235, https://doi.org/10.1542/peds.2018-3835.
4. Lianne Soller, Moshe Ben-Shoshan, Daniel W. Harrington, et al., "Adjusting for Nonresponse Bias Corrects Overestimates of Food Allergy Prevalence," *Journal of Allergy and Clinical Immunology: In Practice* 3, no. 2 (March 2015): 291–293, https://doi.org/10.1016/j.jaip.2014.11.006.
5. R. Pawankar, G. W. Canonica, S. T. St Holgate, R. F. Lockey, and M. Blaiss, M., *The WAO White Book on Allergy*, 2013, https://www.worldallergy.org/UserFiles/file/WAO-White-Book-on-Allergy_web.pdf.
6. Australasian Society of Clinical Immunology and Allergy (ASCIA), "Food Allergy FAQs,"n.d., accessed September 27, 2023, https://www.allergy.org.au/patients/food-allergy/food-allergy.
7. I. Asher and N. Pearce. "Global Burden of Asthma Among Children." *International Journal of Tuberculosis and Lung Disease* 18, no. 11 (November 1, 2014): 1269–78, https://doi.org/10.5588/ijtld.14.0170.
8. Centers for Disease Control, "Interactive Summary Health Statistics for Children," undated, accessed September 27, 2023, https://wwwn.cdc.gov/NHISDataQueryTool/SHS_child/index.html.

9. Lucy J. Griffiths, Ronan A. Lyons, Amrita Bandyopadhyay, et al., "Childhood Asthma Prevalence: Cross-Sectional Record Linkage Study Comparing Parent-Reported Wheeze with General Practitioner-Recorded Asthma Diagnoses from Primary Care Electronic Health Records in Wales," *BMJ Open Respiratory Research* 5, no. 1 (2018): e000260, https://doi.org/10.1136/bmjresp-2017-000260.
10. Dhenuka Radhakrishnan, Sarah E. Bota, April Price, et al., "Comparison of Childhood Asthma Incidence in 3 Neighbouring Cities in Southwestern Ontario: A 25-Year Longitudinal Cohort Study," *CMAJ Open* 9, no. 2 (April 2021): E433–42, https://doi.org/10.9778/cmajo.20200130.
11. KFA Online Community for Managing Food Allergies, "The Social and Emotional Impact of Food Allergies," blog, n.d., accessed September 27, 2023, https://community.kidswithfoodallergies.org/blog/the-social-and-emotional-impact-of-food-allergies.
12. Clara Westwell-Roper, Sharon To, Gordan Andjelic, et al., "Food-Allergy-specific Anxiety and Distress in Parents of Children with Food Allergy: A Systematic Review," *Pediatric Allergy and Immunology* 33, no. 1 (December 11, 2021), https://doi.org/10.1111/pai.13695.
13. R. M. King, R. C. Knibb, and J. O'B. Hourihane, "Impact of Peanut Allergy on Quality of Life, Stress and Anxiety in the Family," *Allergy* 64, no. 3 (March 2009): 461–68, https://doi.org/10.1111/j.1398-9995.2008.01843.x; Christopher M. Warren, Ruchi S. Gupta, Min-Woong Sohn, et al., "Differences in Empowerment and Quality of Life Among Parents of Children with Food Allergy," *Annals of Allergy, Asthma & Immunology* 114, no. 2 (February 2015): 117–25.e3, https://doi.org/10.1016/j.anai.2014.10.025.
14. Ruchi S. Gupta, Elizabeth E. Springston, Bridget Smith, et al., "Food Allergy Knowledge, Attitudes, and Beliefs of Parents with Food-Allergic Children in the United States," *Pediatric Allergy and Immunology* 21, no. 6 (August 18, 2010): 927–34, https://doi.org/10.1111/j.1399-3038.2010.01005.x.
15. Robyn Fawcett, Kylie Porritt, Cindy Stern, and Kristin Carson-Chahhoud, "Experiences of Parents and Carers in Managing Asthma in Children: A Qualitative Systematic Review," *JBI Database of Systematic Reviews and Implementation Reports* 17, no. 5 (May 2019): 793–984, https://doi.org/10.11124/jbisrir-2017-004019.

16. Vaida Taminskiene, Tomas Alasevicius, Algirdas Valiulis, et al., "Quality of Life of the Family of Children with Asthma Is Not Related to Asthma Severity," *European Journal of Pediatrics* 178, no. 3 (January 4, 2019): 369–76, https://doi.org/10.1007/s00431-018-3306-8.
17. James D. Doorley, Fallon R. Goodman, Kerry C. Kelso, and Todd B. Kashdan, "Psychological Flexibility: What We Know, What We Do Not Know, and What We Think We Know," *Social and Personality Psychology Compass* 14, no. 2 (2020): 1–11, https://doi.org/10.1111/spc3.12566.

1. Exploring Unhelpful Allergy Parenting Narratives

1. M. Villatte, J. L. Villatte, and S. C. Hayes, *Mastering the Clinical Conversation: Language as Intervention*, Guilford Press, 2019.
2. J. S. Rolland, *Families, Illness and Disability: A Bio-Psychosocial Intervention Model*, Basic Books, 1994.
3. Elisabeth Kübler-Ross, and David Kessler, *On Grief and Grieving: Finding the Meaning of Grief Through the Five Stages of Loss*, Simon and Schuster, 2014.
4. David Kessler, *Finding Meaning: The Sixth Stage of Grief*, Scribner, 2020.
5. L. Tonkin, "Growing Around Grief—Another Way of Looking at Grief and Recovery," *Bereavement Care* 15, no. 1 (1996): 10.
6. S. C. Hayes, K. D. Strosahl, and K. G. Wilson, *Acceptance and Commitment Therapy: An Experiential Approach to Behavior Change*, Guilford Press, 1999.
7. Hayes et al., *Acceptance and Commitment Therapy*.
8. K. Nadeau and S. Barnett, *The End of Food Allergy: The Science-Based Plan That Turns Food into Medicine*, Penguin Young Readers, 2023.
9. C. S. Dweck, *Mindset: The New Psychology of Success*, Ballantine Books, 2006.
10. Dweck, *Mindset*, 6.
11. N. A. John-Henderson, R. C. Wright, K. J. Manke, et al., "The Influence of Health Mindset on Perceptions of Illness and Behaviors Among Adolescents," *International Journal of Behavioral Medicine* 28, no. 6 (2021):727–36, https://doi.org/10.1007/s12529-021-09972-2.

12. Hagar Goldberg, "Growing Brains, Nurturing Minds—Neuroscience as an Educational Tool to Support Students' Development as Life-Long Learners," *Brain Sciences* 12, no. 12 (2022): 1622, https://doi.org/10.3390/brainsci12121622.
13. Rolland, *Families, Illness and Disability*, 127.

2. Recognizing Common Allergy Parenting Traps

1. Jill A. Stoddard, *Be Mighty: A Woman's Guide to Liberation from Anxiety, Worry, and Stress Using Mindfulness and Acceptance*, New Harbinger Publications, 2020.
2. Jennifer L. P. Protudjer, Michael Golding, Marlee R. Salisbury, Elissa M. Abrams, and Leslie E. Roos. 2021. "High Anxiety and Health-Related Quality of Life in Families with Children with Food Allergy During Coronavirus Disease 2019," *Annals of Allergy, Asthma & Immunology* 126, no. 1 (2021): 83–88, https://doi.org/10.1016/j.anai.2020.09.010.
3. T. Weinberger, R. Annunziato, E. Riklin, E. Shemesh, and S. H. Sicherer, "A Randomized Controlled Trial to Reduce Food Allergy Anxiety About Casual Exposure by Holding the Allergen: TOUCH Study," *Journal of Allergy and Clinical Immunology in Practice* 7, no. 6(2019): 2039–42, https://doi.org/10.1016/j.jaip.2019.01.018.
4. Katherine K. Dahlsgaard, Leah K. Wilkey, Shana D. Stites, Megan O. Lewis, and Jonathan M. Spergel, "Development of the Child- and Parent-Rated Scales of Food Allergy Anxiety (SOFAA)," *Journal of Allergy and Clinical Immunology in Practice* 10, no. 1 (2022): 161–69, https://doi.org/10.1016/j.jaip.2021.06.039.
5. Email message to author, January 2025.
6. Hugh A. Sampson, Seema Aceves, S. Allan Bock, et al., "Food Allergy: A Practice Parameter Update—2014," *Journal of Allergy and Clinical Immunology* 134, no. 5 (2014): 1016–25, https://doi.org/10.1016/j.jaci.2014.05.013.
7. Aikaterini Anagnostou, Vibha Sharma, Linda Herbert, and Paul J. Turner, "Fatal Food Anaphylaxis: Distinguishing Fact from Fiction," *Journal of Allergy and Clinical Immunology in Practice* 10, no. 1 (2022): 11–17, https://doi.org/10.1016/j.jaip.2021.10.008.

8. Anna J. Chen Arroyo, Christine Pal Chee, Carlos A. Camargo Jr., and N. Ewen Wang, "Where Do Children Die from Asthma? National Data from 2003 to 2015," *The Journal of Allergy and Clinical Immunology in Practice* 6, no. 3 (2018): 1034–36, https://doi.org/10.1016/j.jaip.2017.08.032.
9. Ruchi S. Gupta, Elizabeth E. Springston, Bridget Smith, et al., "Food Allergy Knowledge, Attitudes, and Beliefs of Parents with Food-Allergic Children in the United States," *Pediatric Allergy and Immunology* 21, no. 6 (August 18, 2010): 927–34, https://doi.org/10.1111/j.1399-3038.2010.01005.x.
10. Roberta L. Woodgate, Marie Edwards, Jacquie D. Ripat, Barbara Borton, and Gina Rempel, "Intense Parenting: A Qualitative Study Detailing the Experiences of Parenting Children with Complex Care Needs," *BMC Pediatrics* 15, no. 1 (2015), https://doi.org/10.1186/s12887-015-0514-5.
11. R. M. King, R. C. Knibb, and J. O'B. Hourihane, "Impact of Peanut Allergy on Quality of Life, Stress and Anxiety in the Family," *Allergy* 64, no. 3 (March 2009): 461–68, https://doi.org/10.1111/j.1398-9995.2008.01843.x; Christopher M. Warren, Ruchi S. Gupta, Min-Woong Sohn, et al., "Differences in Empowerment and Quality of Life Among Parents of Children with Food Allergy," *Annals of Allergy, Asthma & Immunology* 114, no. 2 (February 2015): 117–25, https://doi.org/10.1016/j.anai.2014.10.025.
12. R. T. Brown, L. Wiener, M. J. Kupst, et al., "Single Parents of Children with Chronic Illness: An Understudied Phenomenon," *Journal of Pediatric Psychology* 33, no. 4 (2007): 408–21, https://doi.org/10.1093/jpepsy/jsm079.
13. M. Annelise Blanchard, Yorgo Hoebeke, and Alexandre Heeren, "Parental Burnout Features and the Family Context: A Temporal Network Approach in Mothers." *Journal of Family Psychology* 37, no. 3 (2023): 398–407, https://doi.org/10.1037/fam0001070.
14. Emily Edlynn, *Autonomy-Supportive Parenting: Reduce Parental Burnout and Raise Competent, Confident Children*, Familius, 2023.
15. B. Brown, "How to Set Boundaries—Brene Brown's Advice," August 20, 2013, https://www.oprah.com/spirit/how-to-set-boundaries-brene-browns-advice.

3. Setting Developmentally Focused Allergy Parenting Goals

1. Christopher M. Warren, Alana K. Otto, Madeline M. Walkner, and Ruchi S. Gupta, "Quality of Life Among Food-Allergic Patients and Their Caregivers," *Current Allergy and Asthma Reports* 16, no. 5 (2016), https://doi.org/10.1007/s11882-016-0614-9.
2. D. Mandell, R. Curtis, M. Gold, and S. Hardie, S. (2005). "Anaphylaxis: How Do You Live With It?," *Health & Social Work*, 30, no. 4 (2005): 325–35, https://doi.org/10.1093/hsw/30.4.325.
3. R. S. Gupta, *The Food Allergy Experience: Real Voices, Real Disease, Real Insights,* Createspace, 2012.
4. Ellen Galinsky, *The Six Stages of Parenthood*, Da Capo Press, 1987.
5. American Academy of Allergy, Asthma & Immunology (AAAI), "Food Allergy Stages Handouts," n.d, accessed November 13, 2023, https://www.aaaai.org/tools-for-the-public/conditions-library/allergies/food-allergy-stages-handouts; Scott H. Sicherer, *The Complete Guide to Food Allergies in Adults and Children*, Johns Hopkins University Press, 2022.
6. Brit Trogen, Samantha Jacobs, and Anna Nowak-Wegrzyn, "Early Introduction of Allergenic Foods and the Prevention of Food Allergy," *Nutrients* 14, no. 13 (2022): 2565, https://doi.org/10.3390/nu14132565.
7. Nancy S. Rotter and Michael Pistiner, "Food Allergies and the Teenager," in *Allergies and Adolescents*, ed. David R. Stukus, 153–68, Springer International Publishing, 2018.
8. Frances Cooke, Ashley Ramos, and Linda Herbert, "Food Allergy–Related Bullying Among Children and Adolescents," *Journal of Pediatric Psychology* 47, no. 3 (2022): 318–26, https://doi.org/10.1093/jpepsy/jsab099; Rebecca Charles, Paul L. P. Brand, Francis J. Gilchrist, Johannes Wildhaber, and Will Carroll, "Why Are Children with Asthma Bullied? A Risk Factor Analysis," *Archives of Disease in Childhood* 107, no. 6 (2022): 612–15, https://doi.org/10.1136/archdischild-2021-321641.
9. M. Arain, M. Haque, L. Johal, et al., "Maturation of the Adolescent Brain," *Neuropsychiatric Disease and Treatment* 9 (2013): 449–61, https://doi.org/10.2147/ndt.s39776.

10. Aikaterini Anagnostou, Vibha Sharma, Linda Herbert, and Paul J. Turner, "Fatal Food Anaphylaxis: Distinguishing Fact from Fiction," *Journal of Allergy and Clinical Immunology in Practice* 10, no. 1 (2022): 11–17, https://doi.org/10.1016/j.jaip.2021.10.008.
11. David R. Stukus, ed., *Allergies and Adolescents: Transitioning Towards Independent Living*, Springer International Publishing, 2018.
12. Marta Vazquez-Ortiz, Claudia Gore, Cherry Alviani, et al., "A Practical Toolbox for the Effective Transition of Adolescents and Young Adults with Asthma and Allergies: An EAACI Position Paper," *Allergy* 78, no. 1 (2023): 20–46, https://doi.org/10.1111/all.15533.
13. Aikaterini Anagnostou, Jonathan O'B. Hourihane, and Matthew Greenhawt, "The Role of Shared Decision-Making in Pediatric Food Allergy Management," *Journal of Allergy and Clinical Immunology in Practice* 8, no 1 (2020): 46–51, https://doi.org/10.1016/j.jaip.2019.09.004.

4. Responding Differently to Anxious Thoughts

1. Catherine J. Norris, "The Negativity Bias, Revisited: Evidence from Neuroscience Measures and an Individual Differences Approach," *Social Neuroscience* 16, no. 1 (2021): 68–82, https://doi.org/10.1080/17470919.2019.1696225.
2. Laura Polloni and Antonella Muraro, "Anxiety and Food Allergy: A Review of the Last Two Decades," *Clinical and Experimental Allergy: Journal of the British Society for Allergy and Clinical Immunology* 50, no. 4 (2020): 420–41, https://doi.org/10.1111/cea.13548.
3. Polloni and Muraro, "Anxiety and Food Allergy," 433.
4. Cleveland Clinic, "What Happens to Your Body During the Fight-or-Flight Response?" December 9, 2019, https://health.clevelandclinic.org/what-happens-to-your-body-during-the-fight-or-flight-response.
5. Georgina Russell and Stafford Lightman, "The Human Stress Response," *Nature Reviews. Endocrinology* 15, no. 9 (2019): 525–34, https://doi.org/10.1038/s41574-019-0228-0.
6. Ravinder Jerath, Molly W. Crawford, Vernon A. Barnes, and Kyler Harden, "Self-Regulation of Breathing as a Primary Treatment for

Anxiety," *Applied Psychophysiology and Biofeedback* 40, no. 2 (2015): 107–15, https://doi.org/10.1007/s10484-015-9279-8.

7. Linda Herbert, Eyal Shemesh, and Bruce Bender, "Clinical Management of Psychosocial Concerns Related to Food Allergy," *Journal of Allergy and Clinical Immunology in Practice* 4, no. 2 (2016): 205–13, https://doi.org/10.1016/j.jaip.2015.10.016.
8. Lilian Dindo, Julia R. Van Liew, and Joanna J. Arch, "Acceptance and Commitment Therapy: A Transdiagnostic Behavioral Intervention for Mental Health and Medical Conditions," *Neurotherapeutics: The Journal of the American Society for Experimental NeuroTherapeutics* 14, no. 3 (2017): 546–53, https://doi.org/10.1007/s13311-017-0521-3.
9. Dindo et al., "Acceptance and Commitment Therapy," 548.
10. Steven C. Hayes, Michael E. Levin, Jennifer Plumb-Vilardaga, Jennifer L. Villatte, and Jacqueline Pistorello, "Acceptance and Commitment Therapy and Contextual Behavioral Science: Examining the Progress of a Distinctive Model of Behavioral and Cognitive Therapy," *Behavior Therapy* 44, no. 2 (2013): 180–98, https://doi.org/10.1016/j.beth.2009.08.002.
11. Contextual Science, "The Six Core Processes of ACT," n.d., accessed May 6, 2024, https://contextualscience.org/the_six_core_processes_of_act.
12. Contextual Science, "Cognitive Defusion (Deliteralization)," n.d., accessed May 4, 2024, https://contextualscience.org/cognitive_defusion_deliteralization.
13. Steven C. Hayes, Jason B. Luoma, Frank W. Bond, Akihiko Masuda, and Jason Lillis, "Acceptance and Commitment Therapy: Model, Processes and Outcomes." *Behaviour Research and Therapy* 44, no. 1 (2006): 1–25, https://doi.org/10.1016/j.brat.2005.06.006.
14. Jill Stoddard, *Be Mighty: A Woman's Guide to Liberation from Anxiety, Worry, and Stress Using Mindfulness and Acceptance*, New Harbinger Publications, 2020.
15. Russ Harris, *ACT Made Simple: An Easy-to-Read Primer on Acceptance and Commitment Therapy*, New Harbinger Publications, 2009.

5. Focusing on All That Matters—Not Just Allergy Safety

1. Olga V. Berkout, "Working with Values: An Overview of Approaches and Considerations in Implementation," *Behavior Analysis in Practice* 15, no. 1 (2022): 104–14, https://doi.org/10.1007/s40617-021-00589-1.
2. Lisa W. Coyne and Amy R. Murrell, *The Joy of Parenting: An Acceptance and Commitment Therapy Guide to Effective Parenting in the Early Years*, New Harbinger Publications, 2009.
3. Jill A. Stoddard, *Be Mighty: A Woman's Guide to Liberation from Anxiety, Worry, and Stress Using Mindfulness and Acceptance*, New Harbinger Publications, 2020.
4. Coyne and Murrell, *Joy of Parenting*, 47.
5. Stoddard, *Be Mighty*, 76.
6. Berkout, "Working with Values", 105.
7. Coyne and Murrell, *Joy of Parenting*, 101.
8. Stoddard, *Be Mighty*, 163.
9. Stoddard, *Be Mighty*, 164.

6. Developing Flexible Perspectives on Allergy Parenting

1. Marie Deschênes, Annie Bernier, Chantal Cyr, Alison Paradis, and Camille-Andrée Rassart, "Marital Satisfaction, Parenting Stress, and Family Alliance: Parental Perspective Taking as a Moderator," *Family Process* 62, no. 3 (2023): 1147–60, https://doi.org/10.1111/famp.12812.
2. Åsa Audulv, Kenneth Asplund, and Karl-Gustaf Norbergh, "The Influence of Illness Perspectives on Self-Management of Chronic Disease," *Journal of Nursing and Healthcare of Chronic Illness* 3, no. 2 (2011): 109–18, https://doi.org/10.1111/j.1752-9824.2011.01087.x.
3. Contextual Science, "The Six Core Processes of ACT," n.d., accessed June 24, 2024, https://contextualscience.org/the_six_core_processes_of_act.
4. Steven C. Hayes, Kirk D. Strosahl, and Kelly G. Wilson, *Acceptance and Commitment Therapy, Second Edition: The Process and Practice of Mindful Change*, Guilford Publications, 2016.

5. Louise Boland, Dorian Campbell, Monika Fazekas, et al., "An Experimental Investigation of the Effects of Perspective-Taking on Emotional Discomfort, Cognitive Fusion and Self-Compassion," *Journal of Contextual Behavioral Science* 20 (April 2021): 27–34, https://doi.org/10.1016/j.jcbs.2021.02.004.
6. Russ Harris, *Getting Unstuck in ACT: A Clinician's Guide to Overcoming Common Obstacles in Acceptance and Commitment Therapy*, New Harbinger Publications, 2013.
7. Jill A. Stoddard and Niloofar Afari, *The Big Book of ACT Metaphors: A Practitioner's Guide to Experiential Exercises and Metaphors in Acceptance and Commitment Therapy*, New Harbinger Publications, 2014.
8. Stoddard and Afari, *The Big Book of ACT Metaphors*, 109.
9. Self-Compassion, "What Is Self-Compassion?," https://self-compassion.org/the-three-elements-of-self-compassion-2/.
10. Kristin Neff, *Fierce Self-Compassion: How Women Can Harness Kindness to Speak Up, Claim Their Power, and Thrive*, Harper, 2021.
11. Neff, *Fierce Self-Compassion*, 25.
12. Neff, *Fierce Self-Compassion*, 26.
13. Koa Whittingham and Lisa Coyne, *Acceptance and Commitment Therapy: The Clinician's Guide for Supporting Parents*, Academic Press, 2019.

RESOURCES

ALLERGY-SPECIFIC RESOURCES MENTIONED IN THIS BOOK

- *The Complete Guide to Food Allergies in Adults and Children* by Scott Sicherer, MD
- *Allergies and Adolescents: Transitioning Towards Independent Living* edited by David Stukus, MD
- *The End of Food Allergy* by Kari Nadeau, MD
- American Academy of Allergy, Asthma & Immunology's "Food Allergy Ages and Stages Handouts"
- European Academy of Allergy and Clinical Immunology's position paper on "A Practical Toolbox for the Effective Transition of Adolescents and Young Adults with Asthma and Allergies"
- Scale of Food Allergy Anxiety (SOFAA) screening tool for practitioners

MINDFULNESS, ACT-SPECIFIC, AND PARENTING RESOURCES MENTIONED IN THIS BOOK

- *Autonomy-Supportive Parenting* by Emily Edlynn, PhD
- *Be Mighty: A Woman's Guide to Liberation from Anxiety, Worry, and Stress Using Mindfulness and Acceptance* by Jill Stoddard, PhD

- *Fierce Self-Compassion: How Women Can Harness Kindness to Speak Up, Claim Their Power, and Thrive* by Kristin Neff, PhD
- *The Joy of Parenting: An Acceptance and Commitment Therapy Guide to Effective Parenting in the Early Years* by Lisa Coyne, PhD, and Amy Murrell, PhD

EVIDENCE-BASED INFORMATION AND EDUCATION RESOURCES

Below is a list of reputable websites offering evidence-based allergic disease information. In addition to medical information, these professional and advocacy/education organizations offer guidance for living with allergies across various ages and stages and information focused on the impact that allergic diseases have on mental health and well-being.

Allergic Disease Information & Allergist Locators

- American Academy of Allergy, Asthma & Immunology: www.aaaai.org
- American College of Allergy, Asthma, & Immunology: www.acaai.org
- Canadian Society of Allergy & Clinical Immunology: www.csaci.ca
- British Society of Allergy & Clinical Immunology: www.bsaci.org
- European Academy of Allergy & Clinical Immunology: www.eaaci.org

- Australasian Society of Clinical Immunology & Allergy: www.allergy.org.au

Allergic Disease Advocacy and Education Organizations

- Food Allergy Research & Education (FARE): www.foodallergy.org
- Allergy & Asthma Network: www.allergyasthmanetwork.org
- National Eczema Association: www.nationaleczema.org
- International FPIES Association: www.fpies.org
- Food Allergy Canada: www.foodallergycanada.ca
- Anaphylaxis UK: www.anaphylaxis.org.uk
- Allergy & Anaphylaxis Australia: www.allergyfacts.org.au

ALLERGY ANXIETY, MINDSET, EDUCATION, AND PARENTING RESOURCES

These resources offer additional tips for addressing the anxiety and overwhelm related to living with food allergies and/or educating children and teens about navigating life with food allergies.

- The Food Allergy Counselor website: www.FoodAllergyCounselor.com
- "Exploring Food Allergy Families," podcast hosted by Tamara Hubbard, MA, LCPC
- "Food Allergy and Your Kiddo," podcast hosted by Alice Hoyt, MD

- *Allergic Living Magazine*'s "Food Allergy Anxiety Guide"
- *Beyond the Allergy Diagnosis: A Guide to Navigating and Understanding the Emotional and Psychological Phases of Allergies* by Simone Albert
- *The Land of Can* book series for children by Riya Jain and J. J. Vulopas
- *A Kids Book About Food Allergies* by Ina K. Chung
- *Wally the Seafood-Allergic Walrus* by Alice Hoyt, MD
- *Not Today, Butterflies! A Book About Food Allergy Anxiety* by Nicole Ondatje
- *My Year of Epic Rock* by Andrea Pyros
- *Zippy: A Story About Oral Immunotherapy (OIT) for Kids* by Sakina Bajowala, MD

MINDFULNESS, ACCEPTANCE AND ACT-BASED WORKBOOKS

While not allergy-specific, these resources can help your family continue to learn and build mindfulness and acceptance skills, which can then be utilized to help navigate the anxiety and overwhelm related to living with allergies.

- *Listening to My Body* by Gabi Garcia
- *The ACT Workbook for Kids: Fun Activities to Help You Deal with Worry, Sadness, and Anger Using Acceptance and Commitment Therapy* by Tamar Black, PhD
- *The Mindfulness & Acceptance Workbook for Teen Anxiety* by Sheri Turrell, PhD, Christopher McCurry, PhD, and Mary Bell, MSW

- *The ACT Workbook for Teens with OCD: Unhook Yourself and Live Life to the Full* by Patricia Zurita Ona, PsyD
- *The Mindfulness & Acceptance Workbook for Anxiety* by John P. Forsyth, PhD, and Georg H. Eifert, PhD
- *The ACT Daily Journal: Get Unstuck and Live Fully with Acceptance and Commitment Therapy* by Diana Hill, PhD, and Debbie Sorensen, PhD

BREATHING EXERCISES

Exercises for the Whole Family

These breathing exercises help calm the mind and body and can be taught to even the youngest members of the family. You can find video tutorials for these exercises online. I encourage you to choose which exercises work best for you and practice them regularly so that you're easily able to use them during periods of increased stress, anxiety, and overwhelm.

- belly or diaphragmatic breathing
- box or square breathing
- bubble breathing
- five-finger breathing
- 4-7-8 breathing
- pursed-lip breathing

Mindfulness and Breathing Apps

These apps offer opportunities to practice calming breathwork and mindfulness meditation exercises—some even have sections for children. It's normal for breathing and mindfulness exercises to initially feel hard, or as if they're not working, so the key is to keep practicing, just as you would when learning a new language.

- Breathe, Think, Do with Sesame app
- Calm app
- Oak app
- Headspace app
- Insight Timer app
- Smiling Mind app
- ACT Coach app
- Peloton meditation exercises

LOCATING LICENSED MENTAL HEALTH PRACTITIONERS

When managing allergies and wanting social-emotional support, it's best to look for allergy-informed licensed mental health therapists, counselors, and psychologists. Even so, allergy counseling is a newer (but growing) field, so it's not always possible to locate an allergy-informed therapist in your area. When this is the case, look for licensed therapists whose focuses include helping those with health anxiety, chronic health diagnoses, and/or medical or health-related trauma.

In addition, due to licensing laws, you'll want to locate a therapist in your state/region, as licensed mental health practitioners can work only with those located in the states/regions in which they're licensed to work, even when offering virtual counseling or telehealth services. The resources below may help you locate therapists near you.

United States

- Academy of Food Allergy Counseling's Directory: www.FoodAllergyCounseling.org
- American Psychological Association: www. locator.apa.org
- Anxiety & Depression Association of America: www.adaa.org
- Psychology Today: www.psychologytoday.com

Canada

- Academy of Food Allergy Counseling's Directory: www.FoodAllergyCounseling.org
- Canadian Psychological Association: www.cpa.ca/public/findingapsychologist
- Psychology Today: www.psychologytoday.com/ca/therapists

United Kingdom

- British Association for Counselling & Psychotherapy: www.bacp.co.uk
- British Psychological Society: www.bps.org.uk

Australia

- Australian Psychological Society: www.psychology.org.au/find-a-psychologist

OTHER HELPFUL RESOURCES

- Avoidant Restrictive Food Intake Disorder information: www.arfidcollaborative.com

- Rome Gastropsychology Directory (GI-focused therapists): www.romegipsych.org
- Equal Eats (travel translation cards for dietary restrictions): www.equaleats.com
- Meg Foundation (needle phobia/fear): www.megfoundationforpain.org
- Smile App (for people managing chronic conditions): www.wearesmileapp.com
- Dr. Kristin Neff's self-compassion information and practices: www.self-compassion.org

ACKNOWLEDGEMENTS

In 2020 when a friend suggested I write a book for families managing allergies, I thought "Sure! How hard could that be?" Turns out, writing a book is hard. It's also not a journey you want to walk through alone, which is why there are so many people I want to thank.

First and foremost, I want to thank Johns Hopkins University Press for the opportunity to write this book. I'm so grateful to my editor Suzanne Staszak-Silva for believing that this book needed to be shared with the world and that I was the one who should write it. Her guidance throughout this process made it much less painful than if I had tried to write this book on my own, for which I am incredibly grateful! I'd also like to thank Tatiana Holway for her magnificent editing and Enid Zafran for her indexing work.

Thank you to Jen Chen Tran for opening the door that got this book-writing adventure going. A big thank you also goes to my literary agent, Laura Bradford, and the team at Bradford Literary Agency for all their hard work that led to making this book a reality.

Special thanks to my friend Jodi Shroba, whose suggestion led to the creative title of this book.

To all my friends who supported me along this journey, especially Alice Hoyt, Paige Freeman, Erin Malawer, Kristi Rude, and Emily Vogel—I can't thank you enough! From fielding text messages saying things like "I'm not sure I can do this" to reminding me why writing this book was important, your support was the fuel that kept me going, especially when life got really tough and complicated.

A big thank you to my therapist, Lori Corrigan, whose support ushered me through one of the toughest and most emotionally exhausting times of my life, which made finishing this book unbelievably challenging. Holding space for me and reminding me to practice the very things I teach my clients continues to help me stay grounded and be the me I want to be, and I can't thank you enough for that.

My incredible village also includes the Mastermind group—psychologists Jill Stoddard, Emily Edlynn, Debbie Sorensen, and Yael Schonbrun—a group of multi-talented women and fellow authors whom I am honored to call friends. I am eternally grateful for their guidance, feedback, and laughter throughout this whole process. Special thanks to Jill for responding when I randomly reached out in 2021 to ask questions about writing a book and finding a literary agent and publisher—you helped me feel brave enough to jump into this journey.

My gratitude also extends to all of my clients, whose willingness to be vulnerable and pursue values-aligned changes in life inspires me; friends and families living with these diagnoses; those researching allergic diseases in hopes of making a difference for those living with these diagnoses; allergist and health care friends who support those living with allergic diseases; and my fellow mental health practitioners who are helping to pave the way in the allergy counseling field alongside me.

To my mom, dad, and our family in England—your excitement about this book and your belief in my ability to write it have meant the world to me. I am grateful for your love and support, not only through this experience, but in life in general.

My husband and kids have my deepest gratitude for their unwavering support, words of encouragement, and patience while I wrote this book. You three are my world, and I love you with my whole heart (or as Nanny would say, "I love you a bushel and a peck!").

Finally, to both of my boys—my hope is that watching me on this book-writing journey has taught you that you can achieve any goal you set, even though it may feel impossible at times. Don't let any diagnosis, worry, or fear convince you that you aren't able to live the life you want to live. Most importantly, know that being your mom is my favorite thing in this entire world, and that I will always believe in you and be there for you.

INDEX

AAAAI (American Academy of Allergy, Asthma & Immunology), 33, 76, 94
ACAAI (American College of Allergy, Asthma & Immunology), 33
Acceptance and Commitment Therapy (ACT): acceptance of anxious thoughts, 122–28; allergy parenting traps and, 44; burnout and, 64; cognitive fusion, 120–22; overview, 14–15; psychological flexibility and acceptance in, 30, 158; self-as-context and, 161–63; values and, 39–40, 132; workability, 115–17; workbooks for, 220–21
accommodations for allergies, 7, 9. *See also* school allergy care plans
adolescents and young adults, 91–101; allergy education and management, 95–97, 192–95; conversations with, 100–101; family therapy and, 193–95; goals and tasks to focus on, 92–98; health management and navigation, 97–98; parents' role, 91–92; points to consider, 98–100; risky behavior and, 92, 192–93
advocacy organizations, 219
allergen-free brands, 25
Allergies and Adolescents: Transitioning Towards Independent Living (Stukus), 94
allergies and allergic reactions, 1–19; Acceptance and Commitment Therapy for, 14–15; accommodations for, 7, 9; anaphylactic reactions from, 55–56, 93–94, 99; author's story on, 3–4, 8–9, 18–19, 137–38, 154–55; defined, 5; emotional distress and fear of, 6–7, 9–11; fatality rates, 55–56, 93–94; medications and treatments for, 3–5; myths on causes of, 31–32; outgrowing, 7; prevalence rates of, 5–6; research on causes of, 32–33; school allergy care plans for, 65–66, 88, 176–77, 190; support and resources for, 7–8, 217–24; symptoms of, 3–4. *See also* safety issues
Allergist Finder tool, 33
allergy care plans in schools, 65–66, 88, 176–77, 190
allergy expert parents, 59–60, 62–64
allergy parenting, use of term, 8
allergy parenting goals, 16–17, 70–102; for adolescence and young adulthood, 91–101; allergy care involvement of children, 73; allergy parenting planning and, 199–200; for infancy, 73–79; journaling questions on, 101–2; for middle childhood, 85–91; takeaways, 101; for toddlerhood and preschool, 80–84
allergy parenting narratives, 16, 20–42; allergy parenting planning and, 196–97; growth mindset and, 36, 37*t*; "I Can't Do This" narrative, 33–36, 161,

allergy parenting narratives (*continued*) 169; "It's My Fault" narrative, 30–33; journaling questions on, 42; "Not What I Expected" narrative, 24–27; open mind for new narratives, 37–39; overwhelm and creation of, 22–23; questionnaire responses on, 20–21; takeaways, 41–42; "This Can't Be Happening" narrative, 28–30; values guiding narratives and beliefs, 39–41
allergy parenting perspectives, 17, 154–80; flexibility in, 163–66; gaining perspective to act flexibly, 174–79; journaling questions on, 180; perspective shifting, 156–60; takeaways, 179; tools for developing, 166–73; on who you are as allergy parent, 160–63
allergy parenting plan, 17, 181–205; creating, 196–204; mindful practices for, 189–95; overwhelm, contributors to, 182–89
allergy parenting traps, 16, 43–69; allergy parenting planning and, 197–98; Burnout Trap, 62–64; Certainty Trap, 48–52; committed actions and, 150–51; Comparison Trap, 44–48; defined, 43; journaling questions on, 68–69; Over-Avoidance Trap, 52–58, 58*t*; Over-Functioning Trap, 59–62; Resentment Trap, 65–68; takeaways, 68
allergy specialists: adolescents' allergy management skills and, 98–99; discussing fears with, 54–55, 150, 185; finding, 33, 218–19; knowledge of, 32–33, 76, 185; risk assessment discussions, 54–56, 66, 113; school allergy care plans and, 88, 176; second opinions, 76, 138; in TRACE, 57; trusting, 76, 185
American Academy of Allergy, Asthma & Immunology (AAAAI), 33, 76, 94
American College of Allergy, Asthma & Immunology (ACAAI), 33
anaphylactic reactions, 55–56, 93–94, 99
anticipatory anxiety, 26, 78–79
anticipatory grief, 26
antihistamines, 4, 9
anxiety and anxious thoughts, 17, 103–29; accepting and observing, 122–28; allergic reactions and, 6–7, 9–10; allergy expert parents and, 62–63; allergy parenting planning and, 200–201; anticipatory, 26, 78–79; anxiety triumvirate and, 49; assessments for, 10, 54; avoiding or controlling, 114–17; being present and grounded, 117–19; breathing exercises for, 110–13, 221–22; of children, 56, 83, 89–90; compassionate self-talk for, 155; defined, 106; food introductions and, 78, 83; ignoring, 12–13, 119; inhibiting life experiences, 131; journaling questions on, 129; mind and body, impacts on, 105–10; new developmental stages of children and, 88–89; online allergy groups and, 45; overwhelm and, 183–84; quality of life and, 70–71; resources on, 219–20; safety and, 141–43; Scale of Food Allergy Anxiety, 54; takeaways, 128–29; unhooking

from, 119–22; useful vs. problematic, 18. *See also* allergy parenting traps; cognitive fusion; safety issues
apps for mindfulness and breathing, 221–22
Autonomy-Supportive Parenting (Edlynn), 63
autopilot mode, 122–24, 196
avoidance behaviors: cognitive fusion and, 120, 150; experiential avoidance and, 29–30, 103, 114–15, 150, 157; helpful vs. unhelpful, 57, 58*t*; Over-Avoidance Trap, 52–58, 58*t*, 77, 83, 88, 161, 191

babies, 21, 73–79
behavioral patterns. *See* allergy parenting traps
belief systems, 22–23. *See also* allergy parenting narratives
belly breathing, 110–13
Be Mighty (Stoddard), 49, 136–37
blame, 31–33, 163
book list, 217–18
boundaries, 47, 65, 67
box breathing, 111–13
brain development, 92
breastfeeding, 32
breathing exercise, 110–13, 221–22
Brown, Brene, 67
bullying, 87
Burnout Trap, 62–64

"can eat" food lists, 83
Certainty Trap, 48–52, 77, 191
cesarean section births, 32
children: anxiety of, 56, 83, 89–90; developmental milestones, 51, 72–73, 186–87; food, relationship with, 83; quality of life and, 70–71; safety and, 142–43; scaffolding learning for, 73; school allergy care plans for, 65–66, 88, 176–77, 190; self-advocacy and communication skills of, 86–87; siblings, food introductions for, 77–78, 160–61. *See also* allergy parenting goals
children, involvement in allergy care: adolescents, 95–100, 192–95; allergy parenting goals and, 73; anxiety reduction and, 56; burnout prevention and, 63; committed actions and, 147; emergency medications and, 82, 86–87, 89, 93, 193–95; middle childhood, 85–89; toddlers and preschoolers, 80–82
cognitive fusion: anxious thoughts and, 120–22, 150, 187; perspective shifting and, 157, 160–61; strategies to counter, 121–22; values and, 150
committed actions, 146–52, 202–3
common humanity, 170
Comparison Trap, 44–48
compassion: perspective shifting and, 160; Resentment Trap and, 65; self-as-context and, 162–63; self-compassion, 162–63, 169–73; self-talk and, 155, 169–70, 178–79; social media battles on, 66; in TRACE, 57
Complete Guide to Food Allergies in Adults and Children (Sicherer), *The*, 76
conceptualized self, 162
confidence: Comparison Trap and, 44–45; competence development and, 61; "I Can't Do This" narrative, 33–36, 161, 169; open-mindedness and, 37–39; playdates and, 81; TRACE tool and, 57

control-seeking behaviors, 49, 188, 190–92
COVID-19 pandemic, 50–51

developmental milestones and transitions, 51, 72–73, 186–87. *See also* allergy parenting goals
discomfort, 119, 178. *See also* avoidance behaviors
doctors. *See* allergy specialists
Dweck, Carol, 34–36, 37*t*

eating out, 53, 177–78
Edlynn, Emily, 63
elementary school children, 85–91
emergency action plans: Certainty Trap and, 50; Over-Avoidance Trap and, 56; perspective shifting and, 159, 168; trusting in, 89, 159. *See also* children, involvement in allergy care
emergency medications: accessing, 66; children managing, 82, 86–87, 89, 93, 193–95; defined, 3; training in use of, 35
empathy, 65
empowerment: allergy parenting narratives, 37, 39; "can eat" list, 83; of children, 87; cognitive fusion hindering, 120; information-gathering for, 36; modeling others' parenting approaches, 138; PACED approach, 75; self-talk for, 50, 178–79; TRACE tool, 57; values and, 39–40, 135
End of Food Allergy (Nadeau), *The*, 32
epinephrine, 3. *See also* emergency medications
European Academy of Allergy and Clinical Immunology, 95
evidence-based information: allergy parenting perspectives and, 175; lived experience-based information vs., 46–47, 185; online information searches vs., 76; resources for, 94–95, 205, 218–19; school allergy care plans and, 176–77; shared decision-making approach, 98–99; websites for, 218–19. *See also* allergy specialists
exercises: on allergy parenting self-description, 164–66; breathing, 110–13, 221–22; on language and tone, 168–69; on mindfulness, 118–19, 125–28; on AND vs. OR mindset, 143–46, 145*t*; on perspective shifting, 158–60; on self-compassion, 172–73; on workability of controlling thoughts, 116
exhaustion, 48, 62–63, 67, 109
experiential avoidance, 29–30, 103, 114–15, 150, 157

Families, Illness, and Disability (Rolland), 22, 39
family mantras, 148–49
family values, 139. *See also* values
fatality rates, 55–56, 93–94
fear: discussing with allergy specialists, 54–55, 150, 185; infants and allergy diagnoses, 74–75; inhibiting meaningful life experiences, 131; in language choices, 167; Over-Avoidance Trap and, 52–58, 58*t*; overwhelm and, 183–84; physiological reaction to, 109; values and, 136, 150. *See also* anxiety and anxious thoughts

Fierce Self-Compassion (Neff), 170–71
fight or flight response, 109, 183–84
Five Stages of Grief (Kubler-Ross), 26–27
fixed vs. growth mindset, 35–36, 37*t*, 157
flexibility: committed actions and, 147, 151; in language choices, 167–69; perspective shifting for, 174–79; values and, 40–41, 137. *See also* psychological flexibility
Food Allergy Counselor website, 205
"Food Allergy Stages Handout" (AAAAI), 76, 94
food challenges, 77–78, 113, 138
food introductions, 77–78, 83, 160–61
food lists, 83
food manufacturers, 25, 45, 49–50
food protein-induced enterocolitis (FPIES), 23
formula feeding, 32

Galinsky, Ellen, 72
genetics, 32–33
goals. *See* allergy parenting goals
Goldilocks Principle, 71
gratitude, 67
grief and loss, 25–27, 75
grocery shopping, 25, 45, 49–50
Growing Around Grief model (Tonkin), 27
growth vs. fixed mindset, 35–36, 37*t*, 157
guilt, 31–33, 162–63, 171

health management and navigation skills, 97–98. *See also* children, involvement in allergy care
helplessness, 28
Herbert, Linda, 112
high schoolers. *See* adolescents and young adults
Hoyt, Alice, 54

"I Can't Do This" narrative, 33–36, 161, 169
infants, 73–79
information: from allergy specialists, 32–33, 76, 185; Comparison Trap and, 44–45; conflicting, 46–47; empowerment through, 36; lived experience-based, 46–47, 185; from online allergy groups, 11, 44–47, 75, 185; overwhelm from, 45, 48, 75–76; uncertainty from lack of, 184–85. *See also* evidence-based information
internal narratives, 22–23. *See also* allergy parenting narratives
International Study of Asthma and Allergies in Childhood (ISAAC), 5–6
internet. *See* social media
isolation, 40, 63
"It's My Fault" narrative, 30–33

journaling prompts: on allergy parenting goals, 101–2, 199–200; on allergy parenting narratives, 42, 196–97; on allergy parenting perspectives, 180; on allergy parenting planning, 196–204; on allergy parenting traps, 68–69, 197–98; on anxious thoughts, 129, 200–201; on committed action, 202–3; importance of, 17–18; on perspective shifting, 203–4; on risk assessment, 198–99; on values, 153, 201–2

Kessler, David, 27
Kubler-Ross, Elisabeth, 26–27

label-reading and labeling laws, 49–50
language and tone, 166–67
lived experience-based information, 46–47, 185

mantras, 148–49
marital relationships, 28, 59–60, 147, 157. *See also* allergy parenting goals; parent conversations
maternal diet during pregnancy and breastfeeding, 32
medications. *See* emergency medications
mental appreciation, 121
mental health disorders, 112
middle school children, 85–91
mindfulness: acceptance and observation of thoughts, 122–28; allergy parenting plan, 196–204; apps for, 221–22; defined, 170; of language and tone, 167; neuroplasticity and, 36; overwhelm and, 189–95; present as focus, 117–20; self-compassion and, 170; unhooking from anxious thoughts, 120–22; workbooks on, 220–21. *See also* Acceptance and Commitment Therapy
mindset. *See* positive mindset
Mindset: The New Psychology of Success (Dweck), 35
mold exposure, 7

Nadeau, Kari, 32
narratives, 22–23. *See also* allergy parenting narratives
Neff, Kristin, 170–71
negativity bias, 104–5, 156, 158–60
neuroplasticity, 36
note-taking. *See* journaling prompts
"Not What I Expected" narrative, 24–27

online allergy groups, 11, 44–47, 75, 185
open-mindedness, 37–39, 66
oral immunotherapy, 113
Over-Avoidance Trap: infants and parenting goals, 77; middle childhood and parenting goals, 88; mindful allergy parenting planning and, 191; overview, 52–58, 58*t*; perspective shifting and, 161; toddlers and parenting goals, 83
Over-Functioning Trap: adolescents and parenting goals, 193; burnout and, 63; infants and parenting goals, 77; overview, 59–62; toddlers and parenting goals, 83
overwhelm: anticipatory anxiety and, 78; contributors to, 182–89; infant allergy diagnosis and, 74–75, 77; information overload and, 45, 48, 75–76; inhibiting life experiences, 131; making sense of, 22–23; mindful practices for, 189–95; PACED approach for, 75–76; resources for, 219–20; "This Can't Be Happening" narrative and, 28–30. *See also* anxiety and anxious thoughts

PACED approach, 75–76
parent conversations: on adolescents and allergy parenting goals, 100–101; on infants and

allergy parenting goals, 79; on middle childhood and allergy parenting goals, 90–91; on toddlers and allergy parenting goals, 84
parenting: allergy expert parents, 59–60, 62–64; stages of, 72; values and, 138–39. *See also headings at* allergy parenting; marital relationships
peer pressure, 93
perspective shifting, 156–60, 203–4. *See also* allergy parenting perspectives; allergy parenting plan
playdates and social outings, 81–82, 103, 190–91
positive mindset: advice for, 38–39; growth vs. fixed mindset and, 34–36, 37*t*, 157; neuroplasticity and, 36; values exercise, 143–46, 145*t*
"A Practical Toolbox for the Effective Transition of Adolescents and Young Adults with Asthma and Allergies" (European Academy of Allergy and Clinical Immunology), 95
preschoolers, 80–84
psychological flexibility: acceptance of emotions and, 30; benefits of, 15; cognitive fusion hindering, 120; defined, 15; mindfulness and, 117; overwhelm and, 182; perspective shifting and, 157–58; safety and, 141–42

quality of life, 6–8, 54, 63, 70–71

relaxed readiness, 15, 71, 110, 182–83, 186–87
Resentment Trap, 65–68
resilience, 35–36, 90, 170
resources, 217–24; on anxiety and mindset, 219–20; books, 217–18; breathing exercises, 221–22; evidence-based information, 94–95, 205, 218–19; for finding allergy specialists, 33, 218–19; for finding therapists, 222–23; increase in, 7–8; websites, 218–19; workbooks, 220–21
restaurants, 53, 177–78
risk assessments, 54–56, 66, 113, 198–99
risky behaviors, 92, 192–93
Rolland, John, 22, 39

safety issues: AND vs. OR mindset exercise, 143–46, 145*t*; anxiety as response to, 104–8; dedicated allergen-free brands, 25; high alert for, 29 negativity bias and, 104–5, 156, 158–60; overdoing it and unrealistic rules for, 21, 26, 40; responding to allergic reactions, 33–34; risk assessments for, 54–56, 66, 113, 198–99; risky behaviors, 92, 192–93; school allergy care plans for, 65–66, 88, 176–77, 190; self-blame and, 31–33; siblings, food introductions for, 77–78, 160–61; sports, 88–89; travel, 88–89, 125, 130–31, 151–52, 177–78; values and, 40, 136, 139–43. *See also* allergy parenting traps; avoidance behaviors; children, involvement in allergy care
scaffolding, 73
Scale of Food Allergy Anxiety (SOFAA), 54
school allergy care plans, 65–66, 88, 176–77, 190

self-administered epinephrine devices, 3. *See also* emergency medications
self-as-context, 161–63
self-blame, 31–33, 163
self-care, 171
self-compassion, 162–63, 169–73
self-kindness, 170
self-observation exercise, 164–66
self-talk: compassion and, 155, 169–73, 178–79; empowerment and, 50; language used for, 166–67; mindset changes and, 36
shame and guilt, 31–33, 162–63, 171
shared decision-making, 98–99
siblings, food introductions for, 77–78, 160–61
Sicherer, Scott, 76
social media: avoidance behaviors and, 29; breaks from, 47; compassion battles, 66; online allergy groups, 11, 44–47, 75, 185
social outings, 81–82, 103, 190–91
SOFAA (Scale of Food Allergy Anxiety), 54
sports, 88–89
square breathing, 111–13
Stoddard, Jill, 49, 136–37, 150
stress: Burnout Trap and, 62–64; chronic and long-term, 109–10; fight or flight response to, 109, 183–84; overwhelm and, 22–23; perspective shifting and, 157; quality of life and, 71; Resentment Trap and, 65; triggers, 64
Stukus, David, 54, 94
sublingual immunotherapy, 113
support: allergy specialists, discussing fears with, 54–55, 150, 185; Burnout Trap and, 62–64; marital relationships, 28, 59–60, 147, 157; networks for, 76–77, 82; online allergy groups, 11, 44–47, 75, 185; Resentment Trap and, 65–68; therapy, 112, 222–23
survival instinct, 29, 105

teenagers. *See* adolescents and young adults
therapy and therapists, 112, 222–23. *See also* Acceptance and Commitment Therapy
"This Can't Be Happening" narrative, 28–30
toddlers, 80–84
Tonkin, Lois, 27
TRACE, 57
travel, 88–89, 125, 130–31, 151–52, 177–78
trust: adolescents and, 93; in allergy specialists, 76, 185; committed actions and, 147; in emergency action plans, 89, 159; in oneself, 31; in others' ability to care for child, 83; Over-Functioning Trap and, 59–62

uncertainty: Certainty Trap, 48–52, 77, 191; lack of information and clarity, 184–85; overwhelm and, 184

values, 17, 130–53; ACT and, 39–40, 132; allergy parenting narratives based on, 39–41; allergy parenting planning and, 195, 201–3; barriers to action, 149–52; clarification exercise, 136–39; committed actions and, 146–49; conflicts and imbalances of, 140–41; flexibility and, 40–41, 137; journaling questions on, 153; list, 133–34; AND mindset exercise, 143–46, 145*t*; overview, 132–36; overwhelm

and lack of connection with, 188–89; safety and, 139–43; takeaways, 152–53
values cheat sheet, 148

website list, 218–19
"what if" ruminations and thoughts, 78–79, 94, 168
workability, 115–17
worry. *See* anxiety and anxious thoughts
worst-case scenarios, 104–5, 156, 158–60, 190

young adults. *See* adolescents and young adults

ABOUT THE AUTHOR

Tamara Hubbard, MA, LCPC is a licensed clinical professional counselor and family therapist with more than 20 years of clinical experience. In her private practice, she provides evidence-based therapeutic support for women, mothers, and parents of those managing allergic diseases. Regarded as a thought leader within the allergy community, she is the founder of the *Academy of Food Allergy Counseling* and its allergy-informed therapist directory. A speaker at national conferences for both patient and practitioner communities, Tamara also created *The Food Allergy Counselor* resource website, which offers evidence-based food allergy mental health, anxiety management, and parenting content, including articles, handouts, and podcast episodes. Additionally, she is an active allied health member of the American Academy of Allergy, Asthma, and Immunology (AAAAI) and the American College of Allergy, Asthma, and Immunology (ACAAI). You can find Tamara on social media at @FoodAllergyCounselor and @TherapistTamara.